Autism

Heartfelt Thoughts from Mothers

by Judy Lynne

Autism Enhancement Publications
P.O. Box 3141, Olathe, KS 66063

ISBN: 1-883175-08-9

First Autism Enhancement Publications printing, January 2005
Edited by *Dan Miller & Diane Speet*

For information regarding special discounts for bulk purchases or fund-raising purposes, please contact Judy@AutismThoughts.com

Cover photo by *Brennan Bargerstock*

Printed in the U.S.A.
Allen Press, Lawrence, Kansas

Dedication

I dedicate this book to all of the moms who trusted me with their most heartfelt thoughts. Thank you so much! I am amazed at all of you who felt called to respond to my email in putting this book together. The only qualification I needed was being a mom to a child with autism and having a heart that wanted to reach out and bring us together, and at the same time, touch the lives of so many others. We did this together because people need to hear 'our voice' and our need to share merely a glimpse of what 'our world' is really like. From Alaska to Texas, Florida to New York, to Finland, Australia, and everywhere inbetween — we are all in this together. We will fight the fight, we will love and let go, we will stay strong and never give up. We know how to give more, even when we don't think we can. We will always love unconditionally. I wish I could be there to hold each and every one of you when times are tough and when the smallest accomplishments are your proudest moments. We must not allow each other to go it alone anymore. Miles may separate us, struggles may test us, but we are all connected heart-to-heart, child-to-child.

With Lots of Love,
Judy

Acknowledgements

To my daughter, Jill – the road has been long and hard but you can count on me to never leave you! Thank you for teaching me 'that which does not kill us – makes us stronger.' Thank you for teaching me the true meaning of 'Let Go and Let God'. Thank you for bringing me to my knees so that I could learn to pray. Thank you for the strength, compassion, patience and wisdom I possess as a result of having you in my life. Thank you for making me proud to be your mother! I love you, as you always say, "best of all". I have been blessed to be loved by you!

I have hired many respite care-providers and am always amazed by the love, friendship, and dedication most have shown to Jill. I am thankful for the teachers like Carol P., Amy F., Jennifer E., Deb E., and Pat G. who have stood by Jill when times were really tough; who endured the spitting, the hitting, the dropping down and yet still believed in her and did their best to teach her how to 'Be' in this world.

To my son, Brennan, who many times took less because I had to give more to Jill. You absolutely are the best son! You are kind and loving, especially to Jill. It meant a lot to me that you would always bring your friends around her. I know you are sensitive to the pain I have endured over the years with all of the heartache involved in caring for your sister. You are so good at making me laugh.

To my daughter, Marie, whose liveliness keeps me going. You are my sweetness! I remember when Marie was 5-years-old and brought her friend over to visit Jill. She explained to her friend that her sister was with Jenn 'because with Jenn, Jill doesn't have autism'. It was so cute. In her mind, Jill was doing so well with Jennifer that she perceived the autism to be gone.

To my sisters, Diane and Sharon - You both have been there, all hours, every time I have called to cry on your shoulders. I don't know what I would have done with out you two! Sharon, you dropped everything and flew across the country because you knew I was alone again and needed help. You had no idea what my life was like until you lived it with me those few days. You came not knowing how you could help but trusted that, just being there for me, would be enough. That was a great gift to me. Diane, your love and constant positive encouragement kept me going even when I was feeling overwhelmed with this project. You shed many tears in helping me edit this book and came away with a new understanding of what raising Jill involves. Your assurance that if something happens to me, Jill will continue to be cared for by people who love her brings great peace to my heart and I thank you.

To my parents who are watching over us from heaven – I will never forget the day my father sat with me while Jill was getting tests done at children's hospital in Washington, D.C. He sat there and said that he had a good life and if he could give it up to make Jill 'okay', he would. We miss you both so much.

To Danny, God was watching out for me when he sent you back into my life after 22 years! Although autism is fairly new to you there is a calmness and gentleness about you that is refreshing for Jill. Thank you for your unending encouragement and guidance with this book. I would not have done it without you. As your tears flowed reading our *Heartfelt Thoughts*, I knew you understood a part of me so few do. Autism has touched your heart as you have embraced mine. Your love fills my soul. Because you believed in me, I believed in me. I love you!

Foreward

Autism is a developmental disability that affects many of our young children and almost on a daily basis I have an interaction with a child with autism or their parent in my office. In many ways it can rob a parent of the opportunity to enjoy watching their child grow and develop. If you let it.

You can learn about autism by reading the vast medical literature, only to be disappointed by modern medicines inability to cope with both the understanding of the cause and also the cure for autism. We are making strides is understanding the complexities of its origin but to this date because of this vacuum of understanding its root cause many theories exist. The internet dwarfs the medical literature in various theories and we must be careful in our interpretation and adoption of the multiplicity of both the causes and solutions. Since we have a vacuum we are at high risk to be set adrift in despair because of this potential loss of hope. This book is an excellent example of the resiliency of the families even when such a difficult medical illness strikes at the core of ones family.

To really learn about autism one needs to merely read the many examples of the power of love and hope even in midst of difficult times. The families depicted in this book lift us up from the despair of our inability to conquer this problem and shows us how much joy we can have in reveling in the uniqueness of our child. I am the parent of a child who is significantly mentally challenged and was in special education her entire life. When she was diagnosed we cried because our dreams were crushed by the fear of the words "mental retardation". We cried because we didn't understand this illness. We cried because we were afraid of the future for our little girl. We had difficulty visioning our daughter as an adult any different than she was at age four when she was diagnosed. We were wrong. Very wrong. She is now first former graduate of special education to be employed as a paraprofessional by the school district and is a happy and self fulfilled young adult. This is a theme in this book that I see in many of the beautiful descriptions of these children with autism. These mothers have refused to let this disease rob them of the joy of the uniqueness of their child. They have realized that to be a successful parent we need only to have our children be physically healthy and also to be happy. We have to adjust our way of measuring success as a parent and just as importantly judging the success for our children. If a child has a several college degrees, a high paying job, several homes and is not happy or has poor self esteem then as a parent we feel we have failed them.

This book stimulates each parent of a special needs child to advocate with the world in order to ensure the success of that unique child. Be careful to advocate out of love rather than anger. Anger is a cancer that can defeat your goal of helping your child. Hopefully by persistence, knowledge and love the teacher or principal will smile when you approach because they see the love you have for your child rather than the hurt and anger that can so easily pervade your thoughts and actions.

It is a joy to read these stories about these children and realize that the love of this parent is the best healing medicine that we have for this special need. These children, as stressed in this book, need understanding but they also need a parent who sets limits for them and gives them guidance about existing in the real world. It is a book that tells us that even with autism we see these children full of special gifts, not just with special needs. It is a book that tells us we are not alone in our struggles and that every victory, no matter how small, is a victory.

Terrance Riordan, M.D.

Introduction

In the early 90's, I was the president of our state's Autism Society and our brochure listed the incidence of autism at 1 in 10,000 births, meaning 1 out of 10,000 children born would be diagnosed with autism. Now, in 2005, I have seen figures indicating an increase to 1 out of 166 – this seems unreal to me. Yet, I am the mother of a 21-year-old daughter who has autism and in the span of her lifetime I have seen autism grow into an epidemic.

I came up with this idea because I have read so many books about autism and yet have always felt I that wanted something more, something that I could relate with other mothers. I knew how I was feeling and thought other moms were probably feeling the same and perhaps wanted to know the same things I did. I have felt very isolated over the years. I found myself blindly trusting people, professionals, etc., in an effort to find help for my child only to sometimes be left feeling even more alone.

As moms we don't usually have a lot of extra time in our daily schedules. Add on a child with special needs and there is even less time. This book is something you can pick up and read a little at a time and something that could be given to anyone to help them understand better the heartfelt thoughts of a mother of a child with autism.

Nearly 100 moms with children of all ages from all over the United States including Alaska and Hawaii; and moms from Finland, Canada, Australia, Belgium and The Netherlands have taken time to share their thoughts with each other and the rest of the world. I asked each mother to submit their Biggest Challenge(s), Greatest Blessing(s), and Words of Wisdom. Most followed this format, some sent poems and stories.

Everyone was so encouraging and supportive in my efforts to collect their thoughts and photos. I instantly felt a connection with each and every mom who shared a story so similar to my own at every stage of their child's life. In some instances moms have more than one child with autism and my heart goes out to them even more so.

I asked for a picture of the moms with their child and a common theme seemed to be that they were always the one behind the camera! It was incredibly touching to look at the pictures and finally see the faces of all the moms who are usually too busy or too tired to have a photo taken. In putting together this book, I knew that the written submissions would have a profound effect on me but I wasn't prepared for the wave of emotions that hit me as I received each and every picture of the moms. You can see the love these moms have for their children, a sense of pure dedication surrounds them. An indescribable bond. Despite all of the struggles we have faced, each and every one of us has a smile on our face when we are with our children. And this is what I wanted the rest of the world to see — heartfelt moments to go along with their heartfelt thoughts!

You will find every mom's written submission for this book is honest and sincere. I believe the response to this project was so great because the need is tremendous. Sometimes we are so involved with fighting for this or that service, or protecting a son or daughter, or educating and advocating for autism awareness that we don't often stop and share how we are really feeling. And sometimes it is a simple matter of just wanting to be heard, to be acknowledged that having a child with autism brings out our best moments and our greatest struggles. Being able to connect with other moms and know how they are feeling has been very comforting whether it is through this book, through letters, through phone calls or the internet, we can look at each other and honestly say, 'yeah, I know exactly how you feel' and truly know that we are not alone.

Reading each entry was bittersweet for me because they all touched me so deeply but I could also feel the pain and worry some of them wrote about. And even though that is the purpose of this book, to feel connected — I found myself wanting to reach out to each and every mom and comfort them. I had received so many entries that brought tears to my eyes that I often times had to just sit and allow the tears to flow and in that, it was very healing for me. I take great comfort in knowing they all feel exactly like I do – sad, scared, determined, patient, caring, proud and... hopeful.

I asked the moms who wanted to, to include their contact information, email or phone number in an effort to connect us all. Please be respectful of their willingness to make that information available to you. If one is not listed, feel free to contact me and I will connect you.

I hope you will treasure our thoughts and share them with anyone and everyone. Autism is not going away and these are Our Voices – the voices of moms who will never give up on their children, no matter what.

With love and light,
Judy Lynne

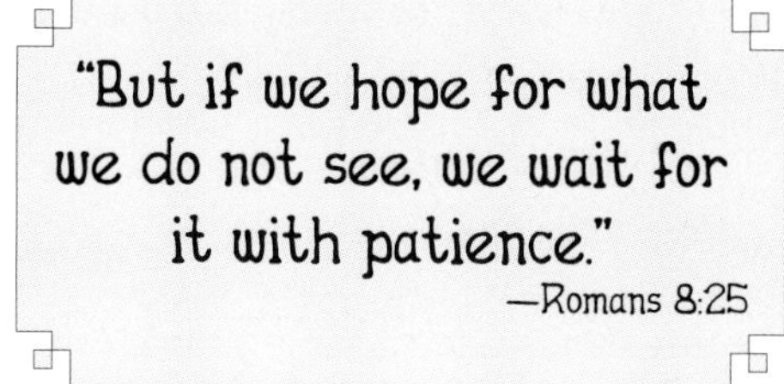

Contents

Contents

Adrianne & Macklin

Illinois

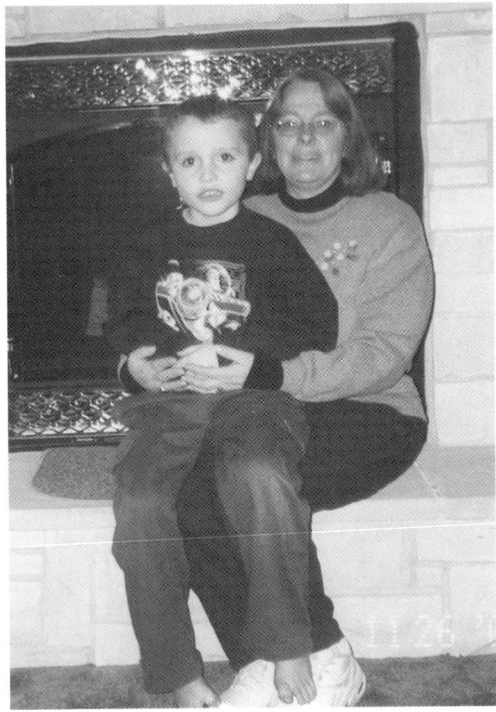

Macklin age 7

Macklin was diagnosed at 3 years

Contact:
847-360-8933
jeffelbe@earthlink.net

Biggest Challenge(s)

My husband. Jeff, and I have been married since 1990. Together we have three children, Evelyn (1995), Macklin (our son with autism, 1997) and Vivian (2000), whom we home school. However, after Macklin was diagnosed with autism in 2000 I was unsure as to whether or not I could teach my children at home. Even though I had suspected Macklin had autism for some time, it was still a shock, and feelings of fear and depression almost overwhelmed me. We had been planning to home school for several years. How could I possibly home school a soon-to-be-kindergartner, a special needs preschooler, AND take care of a new baby? Jeff and I toured our local school district's program. I left the facility in tears, and a new resolve. I witnessed disorganization, chaos, and questionable behavior on the part of teachers and staff towards nonverbal, frightened children. I felt that God was clearly showing me

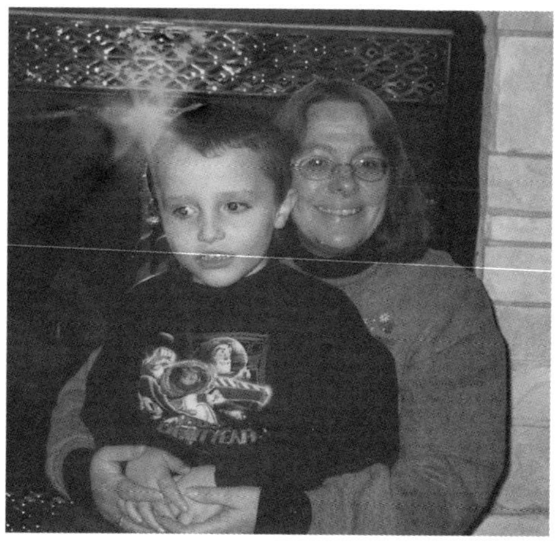

that we were to home school. As I continued my research I learned there is great controversy over the best way to educate children with autism. However, there is one consistent opinion: these children do best in a one-to-one environment, or in an environment which will facilitate this as much as possible. What better place to educate a child with autism than in the home! Our family decided we would rather invest our time, energy and resources into treating and educating our special child at home, rather than attempting to force the school district to do what we felt was best. We feel we have made the better choice. We have been home schooling now since 2000 and have never looked back.

Greatest Blessings

Macklin has brought our family countless blessings. If you had asked me ten years ago if I would have thought I could home school my children, including a child with special needs I would have said "NO WAY!" Macklin has taught me that I have an inner strength and capacity to love that I never knew existed. Because of Macklin I have learned to lean on and trust God, who has given me patience, wisdom and courage. I now understand what unconditional love really means. My idea of "perfect" is also different. I don't see perfection as the world does anymore . . . I look beyond the surface. I used to be a very impatient person. I often say "I prayed for patience and God sent me Macklin." Having a special needs child has also humbled me. Before we had children, I worked in a school for special needs children. I thought I knew a lot, but now I have more understanding, and more empathy and insights. Our family is very close. We rejoice at the little accomplishments Macklin makes . . . the things that come more easily to others. We also do not look back and dwell on "what might have been" but rather look forward to the future with love, hope and trust.

"Because of Macklin I have learned to lean on and trust God, who has given me patience, wisdom and courage."

Words of Wisdom

I would like to address those who are really struggling with their school districts and those who may be considering home schooling. I would like to encourage those families to give home schooling some consideration. Home schooling is a lot of work, but we avoid the stress and hardship of trying to work with an inadequate school system. The energies we would spend on fighting with the school district for a "free and appropriate education" are now channeled towards our son. In the home school, a true Individualized Education Program (IEP) can take place. The family knows the child best and can tailor the learning plan to best meet the needs of the child. Home affords more one-on-one opportunities, and is a safe, loving and supportive environment. Negative peer relationships and teasing/mistreatment are minimized.

Our family is extraordinarily close, and we have witnessed Macklin emerge from a highly anxious, nonverbal toddler to a boy who is kind and affectionate, who is curious about the world and enjoys learning, and who is learning to use functional speech. We see him enjoying life and having fun with his sisters, who love and accept him for who he is. More and more families with special needs children are seeing the benefits of home schooling and are choosing to take control of their child's education. There is support available for those who are considering this direction. May the Lord bless you all as we continue to love and work with our special children.

Favorite Resources:

1) Illinois Christian Home Educators (Lots of support and a page devoted to special needs home schooling): www.iche.org/
2) Five in a Row (literature based unit study we use and homeschool support): www.fiveinarow.com/
3) Do 2 Learn (many free resources and educational tips): www.dotolearn.com/
4) National Challenged Homeschoolers Associated Network: www.nathhan.com/
5) Hope and a Future (the link to Linda Kane, the Neurodevelopmentalist with whom we consult): www.hope-future.org/index.htm
6) *Christian Homes and Special Kids* compiled by Sherry Bushnell & Dianne Ryckman
7) *Home Schooling Children With Special Needs* by Sharon Hensley

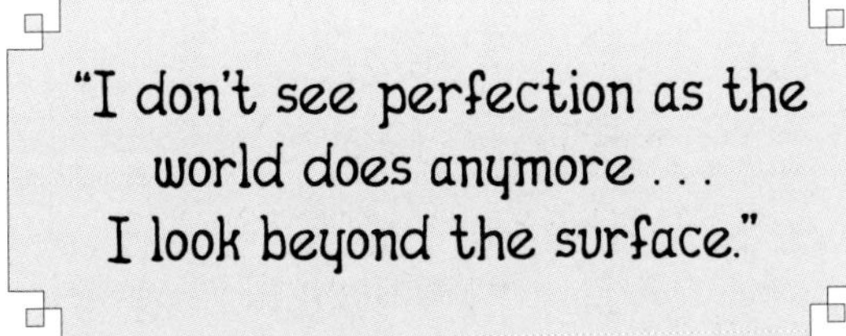

Alessandra & Nicholas

Massachusetts

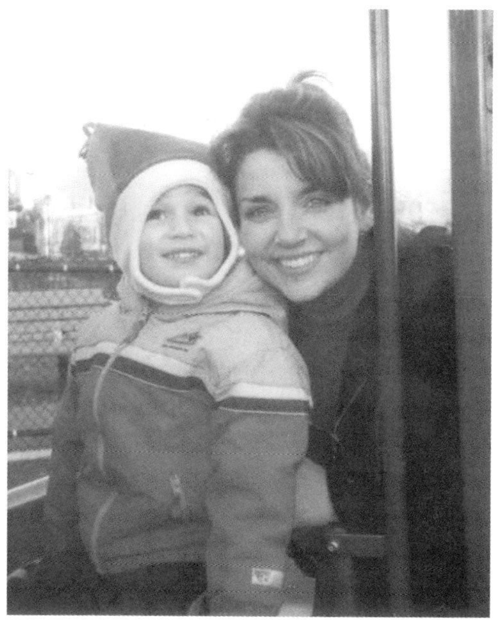

CONTACT:
Kunfoo@aol.com

Nicholas was diagnosed at 29 months

BIGGEST CHALLENGE(S)

I am blessed with a beautiful son Nicholas who turned 4 on December 16th. Nicholas was diagnosed with PDD/NOS (Pervasive Developmental Disorder/Not Otherwise Specified) at the age of 29 months. Nicholas is doing great, becoming more verbal and social and has always been a very loving and funny little fellow. He is the love of my life.

One of the biggest challenges I feel is worrying about Nicholas' future. I think all parents worry about their children's future, but when your child has autism, its even more difficult. You want a crystal ball to just see if they will be able to speak if they are not verbal now. You wonder, "Will they make friends?", "Will people notice they are different?", "Will they work?", "Will they get married and or have a family?", "What will happen when I am gone?", "Will they be cared for and loved as much as they are now?", "Will they be happy?"

Greatest Blessings

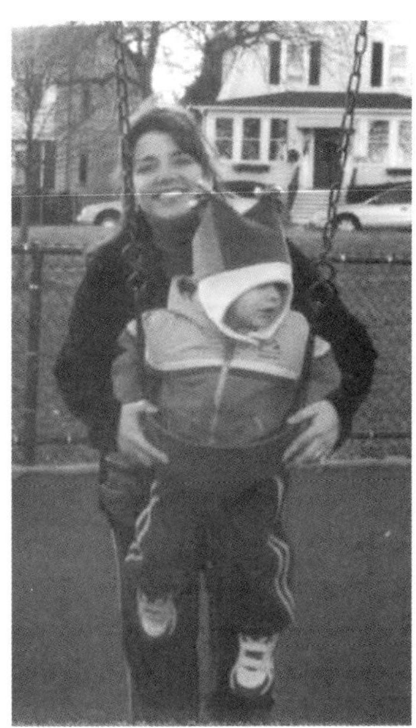

One of the greatest blessings for me is truly appreciating every little thing he accomplishes. All parents are excited when their child says their first word, but for a parent with a child who has autism it's like winning the lottery! The first time Nicholas associated a word correctly I almost burst into tears...he watched a TV show that had a picture of the ocean and looked at me and said "wadder!" He was 3. I couldn't believe it and told my friends who were with us there (with neuro-typical children) and I noticed they didn't realize how huge that was...you'd have to be a parent of an autistic child to really know how wonderful that was.

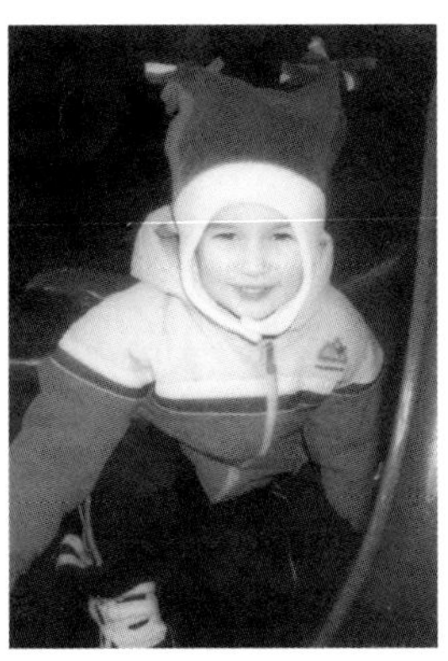

Words of Wisdom

Some words of wisdom I've heard are to educate people on autism. I used to hide it more when I first was dealing with it, but now I try to explain what Nicholas has to others if I see some interest. It helps others not to fear the unknown. I think the more people are aware of what autism is, the better it will be for our children.

Favorite Resources:

Early Intervention and Building Blocks are two services/organizations that really helped in the beginning and gave me a lot of support and knowledge.

> "All parents are excited when their child says their first word,
> but for a parent with a child who has
> Autism it's like winning the lottery!"

Andrea & Monica

Missouri

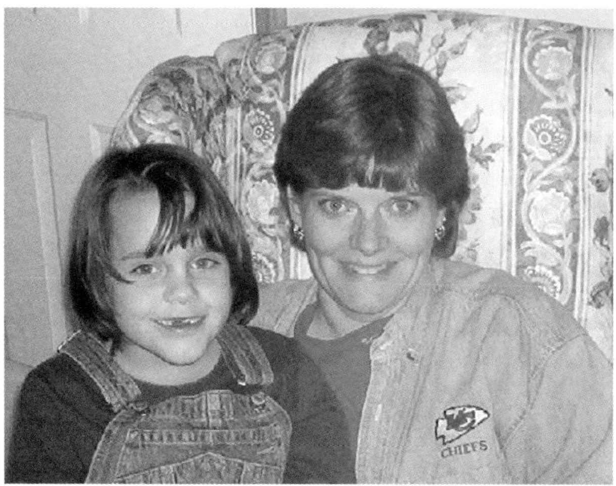

Monica was diagnosed at 7 years

Greatest Challenge(s)

- Fighting for an appropriate education.
- Not getting a diagnosis until the age of seven.
- Getting extended family to except her as she is.
- The amount of frustration Monica carries and trying to help her express herself without melting down.
- Trying to work through literal thinking (ex. Saying good-bye doesn't mean forever).
- Sensory integration – understanding how sensitive Monica can be to certain touch or sounds. Some days you can touch her and it's okay, other days she says "Ow you hurt me!" Monica can be oblivious to pain. She slammed her fingers in my car door and never cried. When I opened the door she said "Oh" and kept on going.
- Discipline – spanking makes Monica laugh or thank us. Time outs are for me.

Greatest Blessings

- Monica has given us unconditional love.
- Monica has taught us the true meaning of patience.
- Small things do count.
- Being potty-trained at the age of six.
- Our church family has accepted her for who she is.

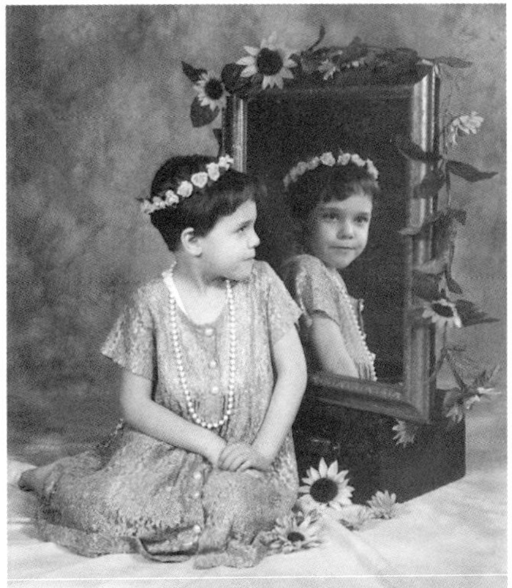
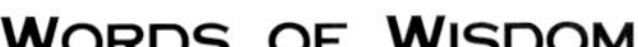

Monica age 6

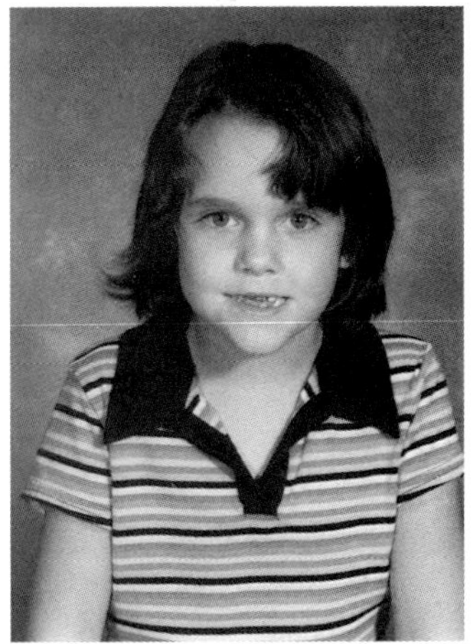

Monica age 7

Words of Wisdom

- Learn all you can, knowledge is power!
- Don't give up.
- Lower your time frame of expectations.
- Remember you are not alone!
- Everyday is a new day.

Favorite Resources:

1) *Your Life is NOT a Label* by Jerry Newport
2) *Thinking in Pictures* by Temple Grandin
3) *Keys to Parenting the Child with Autism* by Marlene Targ Brill, M.ED.
4) *The Out-of-Sync Child by* Carol Stock Kranowitz, M.A.
5) *Emergence: Labelled Autistic* by Temple Grandin

Angela & Danny

Missouri

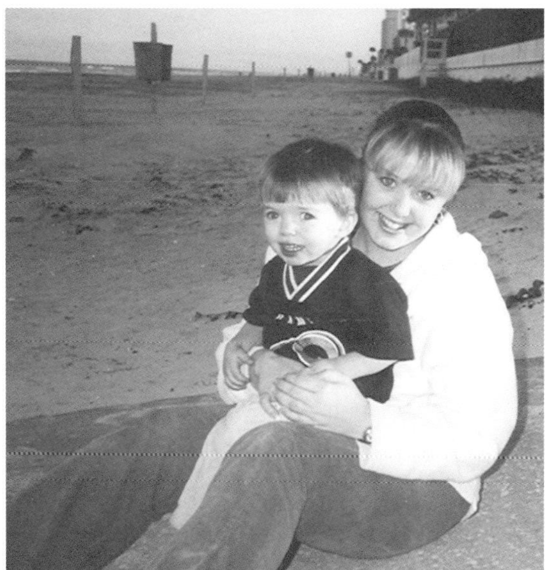

Danny was diagnosed at 2 years old

Biggest Challenge(s)

One of the biggest challenges I face as a mother of a child with autism isn't the school, therapies, or even no communication. The biggest challenge I face everyday is reactions from family, friends, neighbors, and the public. They ask, "Why is he staring at his hand?" or "He's 3 and not potty trained yet?", and my favorite, "Is he deaf?" I respond with, "He's autistic" and wait for their reaction. To me, it's not a big deal. He is a happy, healthy, active toddler who learns at his own pace. I still can't believe the number of people that ask "How did he get it?" or "Will he ever be normal?" I have learned to take that negativity and turn it into something useful such as educating myself or others.

Greatest Blessings

I cannot think of any blessings in particular since my son has come along, because there are so many. He IS my greatest blessing. He came into my life when it was full of chaos and turned it around for the better. He has given me the patience I never had, the confidence I could never find, and makes me want to be a better person. He doesn't care what I look like, what I wear, what I drive, or where we live. As long as his needs are met, he is the happiest person I've ever met in my life. If only more people could be like him.

> "He doesn't care what I look like, what I wear, what I drive, or where we live. As long as his needs are met, he is the happiest person I've ever met in my life. If only more people could be like him".

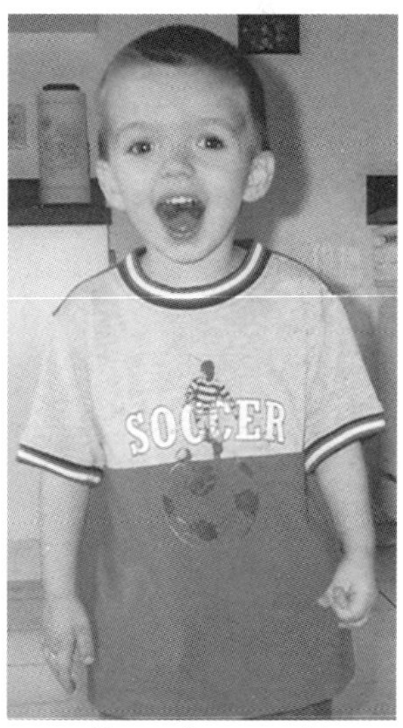

Danny 3 years old

Words of Wisdom

Something that I'll keep with me for the rest of my life happened on the hottest day of the year, inside a doctor's waiting room full of people. My son was sick, and a woman sitting next to us was trying to help me calm him down. As we talked and he cried, she told me her granddaughter had just been diagnosed with autism. I then told her about my son and his diagnosis, and we continued talking for half an hour as we waited. When my name was called, the woman patted my back and told me "God gives special children to special people."

Angie & Michael

Oregon

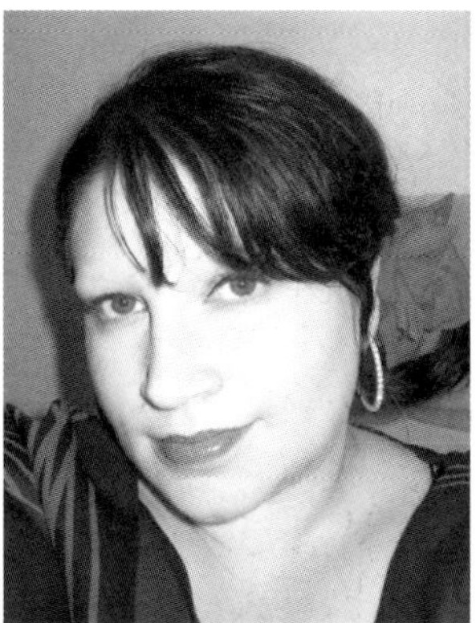

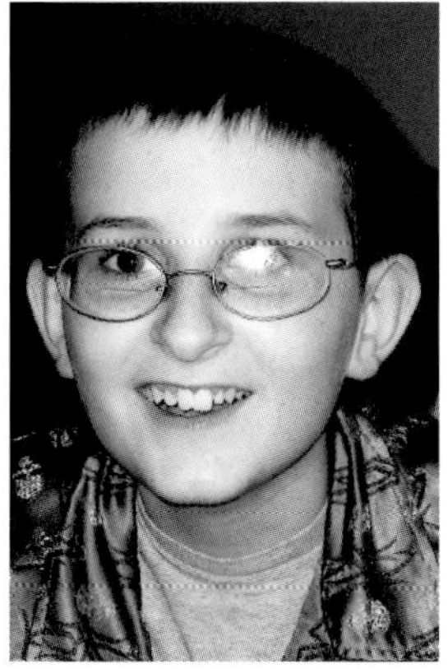

Michael 11 years old

Biggest Challenge(s)

My biggest challenge as Mikey's mom is to try and be patient and understanding ALL of the time. It is an all-the-time job, no breaks and no raises! At times I'm just tired and my brain hurts from all the thinking ahead that must be done day-to-day, to ensure Mikey's days can go as smoothly as possible. It can also be a challenge to get new teachers or care providers to understand in a short period of time what it has taken me years to learn.

Greatest Blessings

There are so many blessings that come with being Mikey's mom. The greatest one to me is that I get to be so close to him. I know many parents who try and be as close with their own children. Mikey's very special mind gives us the opportunity to have a relationship on a much greater level.

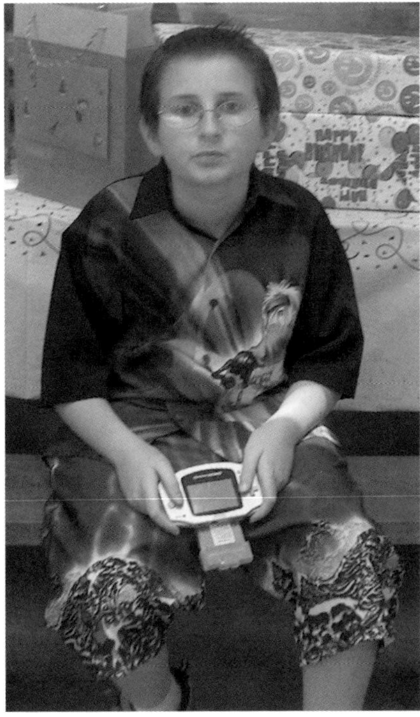

"Everything has beauty, but not everyone sees it."

– Anonymous

Words of Wisdom

My words of wisdom are very basic. Every person, every place, at every moment should just be mindful of our great differences. We should try and accept each person as an individual, and think about what that word really means:

Individual

April & Daniel

Arkansas

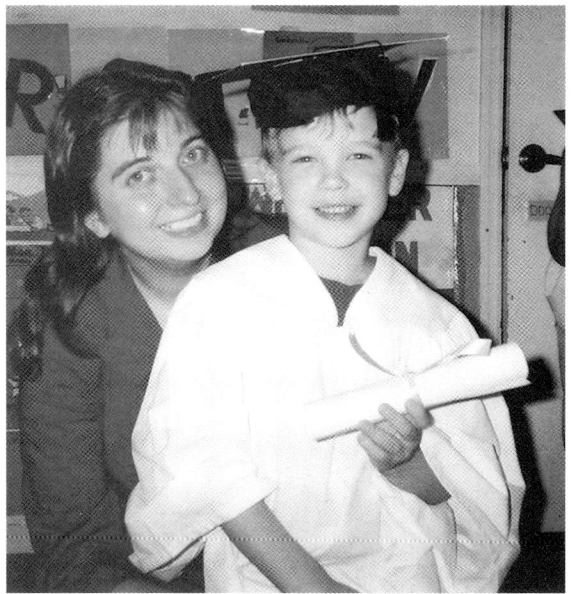

School Graduation 2003

CONTACT:
veronicalee97@yahoo.com

Daniel was diagnosed at 2 years, 3 months

BIGGEST CHALLENGE(S)

The biggest challenge has been a communication barrier. Daniel never seemed to understand what you were telling him. I would describe it as you speak one language, I speak another, and neither of us knows the other language to understand each other. Finally, a year ago, when Daniel turned 6 he started understanding some of the requests I would have for him. Throughout the year Daniel had comprehended more language. Daniel's receptive speech is really improving, but he still has a long way to go with expressive speech. We still don't have "typical" conversations with each other. He is still learning how to do that, but someday we will.

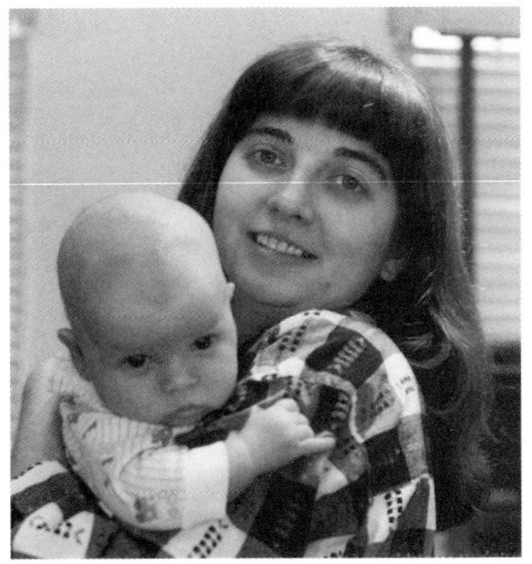

Daniel 1998

Greatest Blessings

It is a great blessing to live in Arkansas, which currently has many educational and financial resources to help children and their families. Another great blessing is having access to parents from many parts of the world through the internet. Other parents sharing their knowledge and resources with me have been my greatest help and support to get Daniel the most help.

Words of Wisdom

Don't let anyone tell you your child will never be able to accomplish something or will never get better. If I had listened to the "professionals" Daniel would not be GFCF, he would still be getting vaccines, he would be taking drugs to calm his behavior, and he wouldn't be chelating for heavy metal toxicity. Search for the root cause or causes of the autism. The best advice I received, when I first learned that Daniel had autism, was from the mom of a daughter with autism. She said, "You will be your child's biggest advocate. There is help out there, but you will have to get the help for your child. No one will do it for you." She was exactly correct. And, that is what I strive to do everyday. It can be stressful work, but the payoff; seeing your child succeed is the greatest reward.

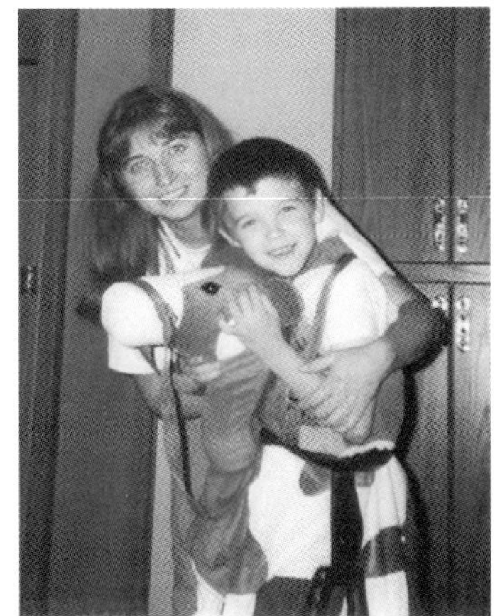

Halloween 2004

"You will be your child's biggest advocate. There is help out there, but you will have to get the help for your child. No one will do it for you."

Belynda & Rebeka

Missouri

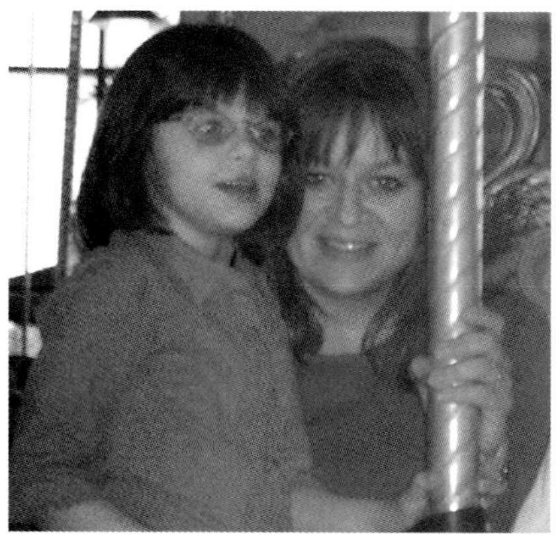

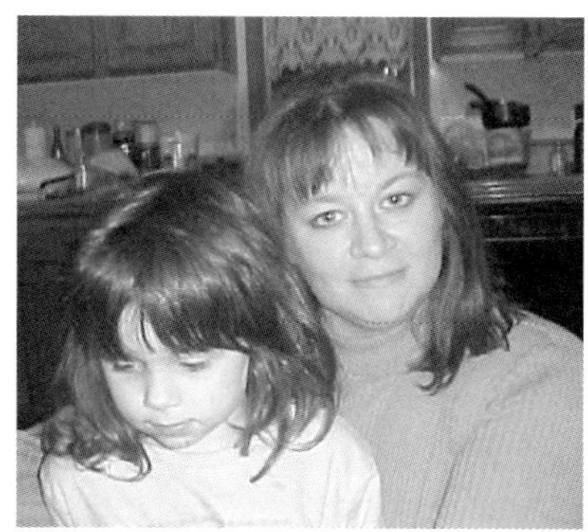

Rebeka was diagnosed at 2 years

Contact:
bfdamiller@hotmail.com

Biggest Challenge(s)

Rebeka was diagnosed at age two. She had several words at 18 months: mama, daddy, baby, ball, etc., but stopped talking around that time. She injured her hand on the treadmill and we thought it had traumatized her so she stopped talking. When she hadn't started talking again by age two, we took her to the pediatrician who had treated her hand and he sent us for a hearing test and a school psychological evaluation. This was in Minnesota where the only required diagnosis for state-funded therapies is a school psychologist. We now live in Missouri.

My biggest challenge with my beautiful daughter, Rebeka, has been accepting her autism. It is difficult to accept, that even though she looks completely normal, her brain is not. Instead of accepting her as she is, I always seem to be trying to "fix" her. I keep hoping for a miracle, even as I try different therapies, vitamins, minerals, diets, etc. Although I keep praying everyday that she will be "cured," I also thank the Lord everyday because Rebeka is such a blessing to me and my family.

Greatest Blessings

Rebeka is a wonderful blessing. She is a very sweet, loving child. Her hugs are the highlight of my day. Everyone I know will do whatever it takes to make Rebeka laugh because her laugh is so pure — never forced at all. Rebeka has also helped me and my family to appreciate every little achievement, every word learned, and every response. Some of my most profoundly thankful moments occur whenever Rebeka makes a breakthrough, big or small.

Words of Wisdom

I don't know if I have any words of wisdom to offer. Just try to remember that children with autism are children. They need love, affection, praise, discipline and kindness just like every other child. Even though children with autism may not show their emotions in typical ways, they are showing their emotions in their own ways and it is up to you to figure out how to decipher those emotions.

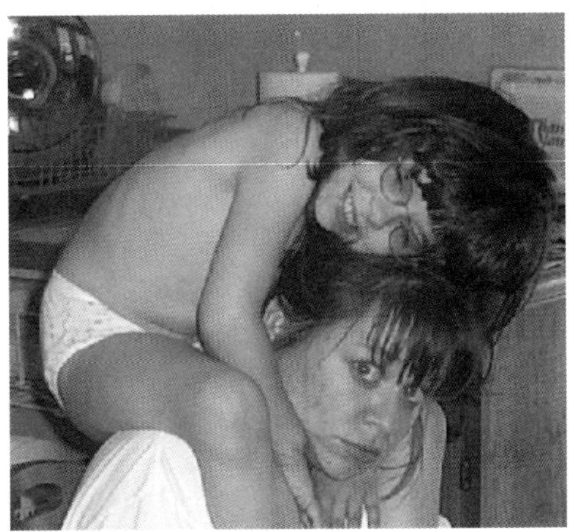

"Even though children with autism may not show their emotions in typical ways, they are showing their emotions in their own ways and it is up to you to figure out how to decipher those emotions."

Betsy & Austen

Georgia

Austen was diagnosed at 3 years

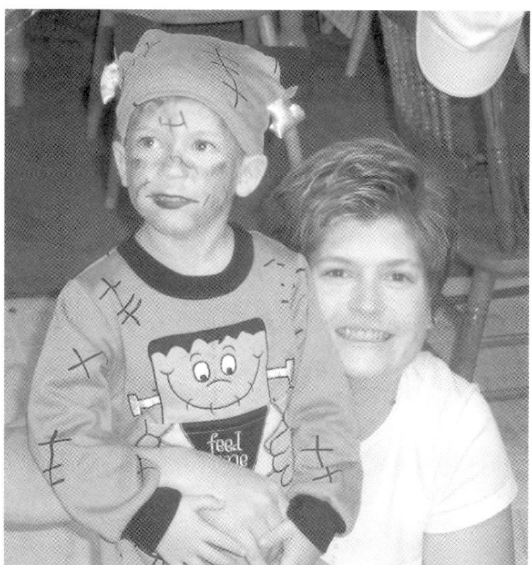

Austen 3 ½ Years

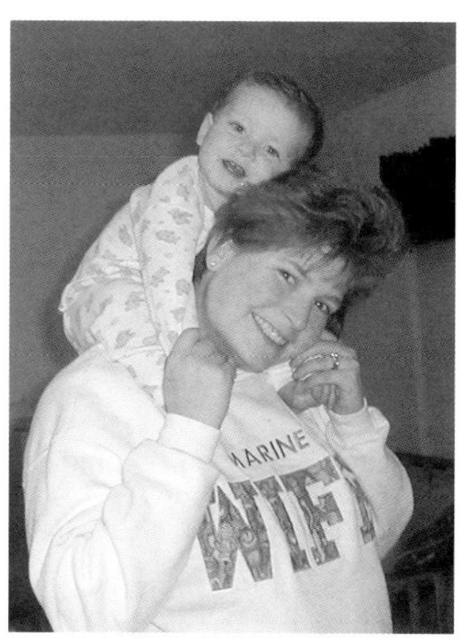

Austen 13 Months

CONTACT:

unlockingautism4austen@yahoo.com

BIGGEST CHALLENGE(S)

There have been several challenges I have faced having a son with autism. To be honest, Austen's diagnosis at age 3 of autism was a relief to me. I knew there was something seriously wrong when he pulled the door off of the hinges in a rage at 18 months, was violent, non-verbal, self-injurious, and destructive. When your toddler's behavior changes so quickly right in front of your eyes, it can be alarming. I wondered what I had done wrong, what had made this happen to my beautiful son? For me, it was not a slowly progressing situation that I just did not notice. My son's behavior changed in a matter of a month. He was talking like a normal 12-month-old, and then he just stopped. He went from hugging me and kissing me, to biting me. I was relieved that "it" (autism) had a name, and made it my mission to understand him and help him. I was so relieved that I did not cause this to happen to him. I buried myself in research, studied the different educational programs, hired every specialist I could, and reached out to as many other parents as I could. I learned how to understand Austen, and why he behaved the way he did. It is really a different way of life. I realized the effort required for Austen to survive in our world. My entire life changed.

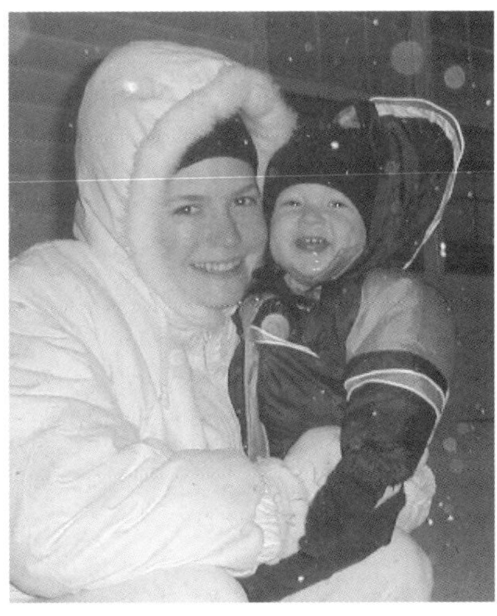

One thing that really made me crazy was when people in public would stare at me and whisper about what a "brat" my child was, and complained about my parenting skills. Once I learned about ASD and that it was the autism and not Austen or me, I started actually giving out business cards that described ASD and gave a web site for strangers to go to in order to learn more. This stopped the dirty looks and rude comments. Once a stranger learned that he had autism, and I handed them a card, the looks on their face were priceless.

My biggest challenge through this entire journey was getting appropriate services for Austen. This is one issue I really feel strongly about. When dealing with the school district I faced adversity in every direction. I wanted an appropriate education for my son, and they refused to do this. I pulled up my sleeves and fought the fight. I am still fighting, it is endless. I am amazed at the lengths some schools will go to in order to deny our children an appropriate education. The obstacles placed in front of us have been numerous. It has been an emotional roller coaster for me as a mom. I am one of the only people who truly understands Austen, and I know what he is capable of. His education is something I feel very passionate about. I know he is very intelligent, and can be a functional adult with the right education and intervention. Unfortunately, there are few educators who really understand ASD.

Being his mother and advocate has been the biggest challenge in my life. It has taught me a great deal about things I never dreamed I would have encountered. It was extremely frustrating and confusing to navigate through the system. It continues to be a daily struggle, but I feel more confident in my own advocating abilities now. No matter how difficult it is, I continue to fight for Austen and his education. Austen needs me to advocate for him so that he may become the functional adult I know he is capable of. So, I gave up my career, quit my job, and started focusing on Austen. He did not have another chance. I was it. Giving up has just never been an option for me. I owe it to Austen, I am his mother.

Greatest Blessings

I have been blessed with Austen. He is a beautiful, smart, and loving little boy. Everything he has accomplished is a miracle to me. He went from being non-verbal to speaking in 6 word sentences by the time he was four. When the right educational program was put into place for him, he just exploded with knowledge. He soaked up the learning like a sponge. It was like he was shouting, in his own way, from a mountain top, "See, I am smart. I can do it! I just needed to be taught a different way." I don't know of a prouder moment than watching my son playing baseball on a field with typical kids and loving the attention and conversation with the other kids. Or, when he made eye contact with me and said, "Mommy." These are little things many parents of typical children take for granted. These are moments that are so precious to me, because I know how hard Austen had to work to accomplish these things. I feel blessed that he is so affectionate towards me. I know that could be different, because it is for so many of my friends with ASD children.

> "Don't beat yourself up. You did not cause this, and you cannot fix it alone."

I feel blessed that I have such a wonderfully accepting family who truly has taken the time to love and accept my son for who he is not the label he wears. I have lost many friends, through this, because they did not understand autism. I feel blessed, though because I found so many new friends who really care about Austen and I and love us no matter what. I found therapists for Austen that have become close friends. I cannot thank them enough for just doing what they do. My son's life has changed because of his Applied Behavior Analysis (ABA) team. We have had to legally battle our school system concerning Austen's educational services. Austen's attorney is an exceptional woman. I feel blessed to call her my friend. It was like God knew what we were about to endure, and put the right people in place to support us through it. The journey Austen and I have walked together has forced me to become more courageous, more humble, and patient. I am thankful for this. I was blessed with a son who has taught me more about myself with each passing day.

Words of Wisdom

I would advise other parents to become very knowledgeable regarding your rights and the rights of your child concerning the law and educational services. It is amazing what schools try to get away with concerning our kids. Another important thing is to remember to take care of yourself. Rest when you have the opportunity. Get out and do things for yourself. Reach out to other parents with children with autism, it can be so helpful and comforting. Always trust your gut instincts. I have found that my gut instinct is usually correct. Think outside the box.

There is a great deal of research and suggestions for children with autism. Not every suggestion works with every child. Sometimes you have to modify or individualize certain things for each child. Read everything you can so that you can be informed about all of the different interventions and educational services for your child.

Lastly, don't beat yourself up. You did not cause this, and you cannot fix it alone. There are so many people going through similar situations, and there are caring people out there who will help. We can all help each other by reaching out and sharing our experiences honestly. Educating others and helping others can only make this journey easier for those whose children will be diagnosed tomorrow.

The Little Yellow Bus

by Judy Lynne, 1987

Growing up in suburban Virginia we had it all, Julie, Kathy, Debbie and I: intact families, the ability to roam the neighborhood without the worry of being kidnapped, enough money to keep up with the latest fads, and parents who made sure we had all we needed. We believed we would grow-up, get married and have kids - the American dream - the perfect world.

But across the street things weren't so perfect. There was that little yellow bus that came to pick up the neighbor boy every day, shuttling him off to school - not our school, a special school. Back then they didn't send disabled children to our schools, perhaps they thought we had nothing to teach them nor did they have anything to teach us... perhaps they were wrong.

Well, my girlfriends and I all grew-up, and yes, we all got married (some of us more than once) and out of the four of us, it was only I who had children. This is when I learned that the American dream doesn't always turn out like one has planned and the world truly is imperfect; not only for the boy who lived across the street, but for my little girl. Next thing I knew that Little Yellow Bus was coming to pick-up my daughter, and Autism became a familiar way to describe her behaviors.

God, forgive me for not realizing that boy across the street had something to teach me back then. For now I know one of the hardest things a mother will do is put her child on that Little Yellow Bus, and the true meaning of the American dream is Unconditional Love.

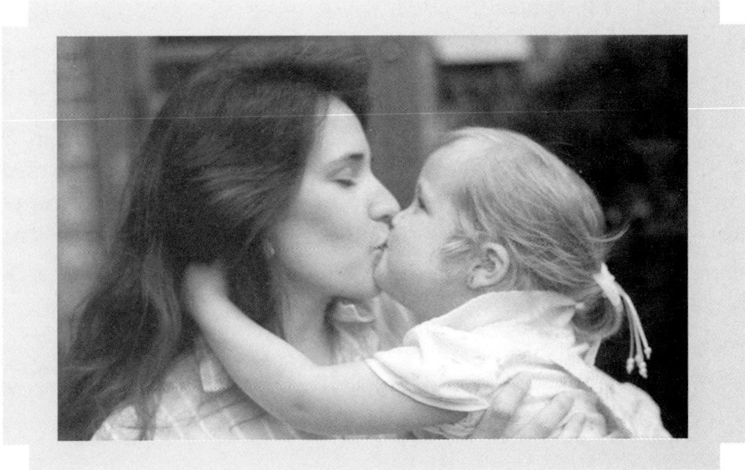

Jill at 3 years old

Betsy & Cammy

Arizona

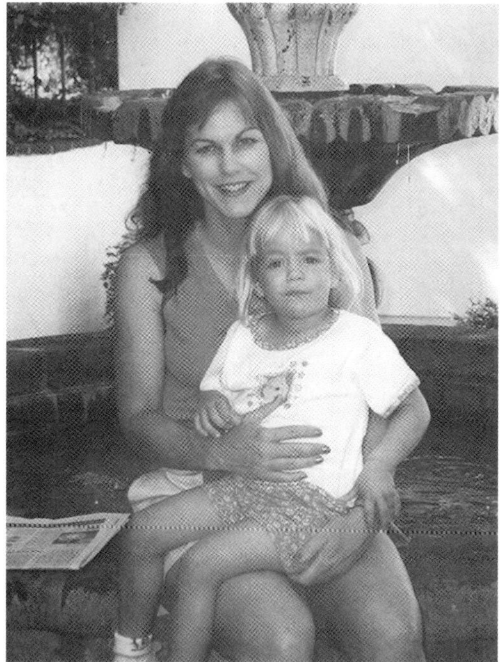

Cammy was diagnosed at 5 years

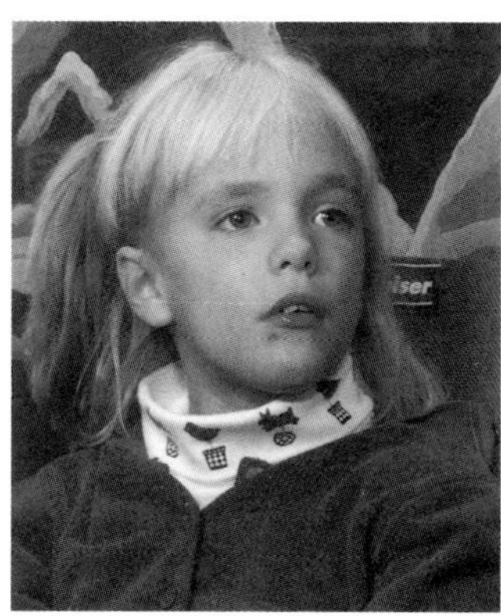

Cammy age 7

CONTACT:
cammye98@yahoo.com

BIGGEST CHALLENGE(S)

The single biggest challenge in being Cammy's parent is not knowing what she wants and needs because she can't talk. It is so frustrating for both of us at times because I can see on her face that she wants to talk, but she can't. When she is sick I have to guess where she hurts. When she is sad I don't always know why. When she is happy or something strikes her funny, I don't always "get it" and she can't share her joke with me.

Another challenge is how much of life Cammy is excluded from. She isn't invited to children's birthday parties; she doesn't have friends come over to play. Even family members don't invite her along on outings with her cousins, such as going to the zoo, parks, movies, etc. So most of the time it's just the two of us going places, which often feels very lonely.

Sometimes the challenge is just getting through the day, or the night (like many children with autism, Cammy frequently has times when she is up at night.)

Greatest Blessings

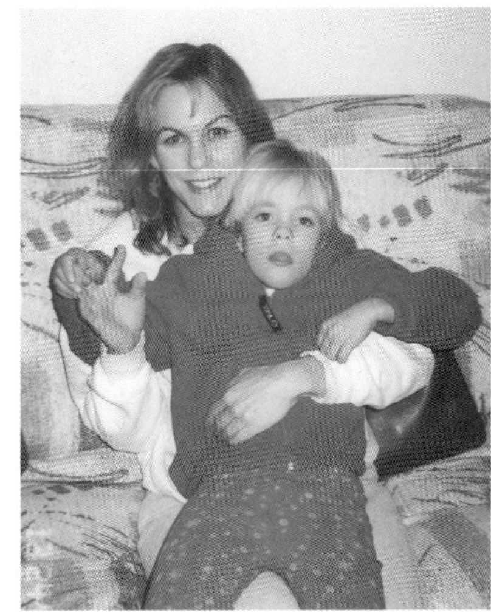

In spite of all the difficulties, my daughter is the greatest blessing in my life. I have learned more from being her parent than I have from any other life experience. I have learned to be more patient, more giving, and to celebrate the small successes in life. Cammy has taught me to look at life differently; she reminds me constantly to be in the moment because that's where she is. Because of Cammy, I know how important compassion and understanding are and how important it is to treat everyone with dignity.

I am also blessed with a supportive family and friends. I don't know what I would do without their help and their willingness to listen when I need someone to talk to. We are also fortunate in that there are some wonderful professionals in Cammy's life who work hard to help her communicate and reach her potential.

Words of Wisdom

When I tried to think about words of wisdom for other parents, the first thing that came to mind was "breathe." Some days I get so tense, between being a full-time teacher and taking care of Cammy as a single parent and juggling respite providers and therapies and not getting enough sleep, and I realize that I need to take a deep breath. Some things I try to remember are: Ask for help when you need it. Take breaks from your child. Trust your heart and feelings. You know what's best for your child. Try to see the humor in situations and laugh everyday. Cry when you need to. See your child for the blessing that they are, not just for the problems that they have. Be their strongest advocate and get them what they need and deserve. Be kind to yourself. Be gentle with people who don't understand. Most of all, be gentle with yourself and your child.

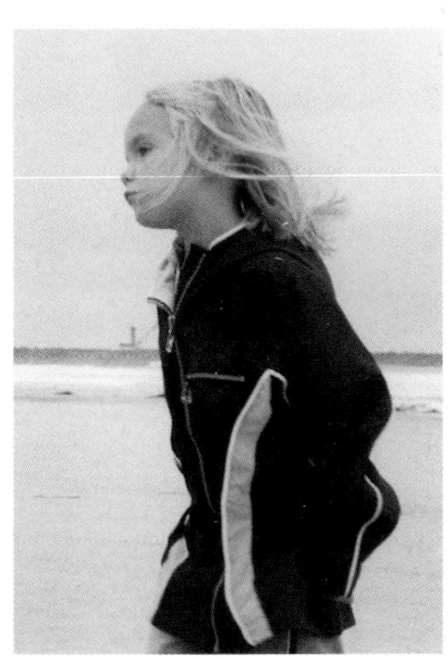

Cammy age 5

> "When I tried to think about words of wisdom for other parents, the first thing that came to mind was 'breathe.'"

Beverly & Andrew

North Carolina

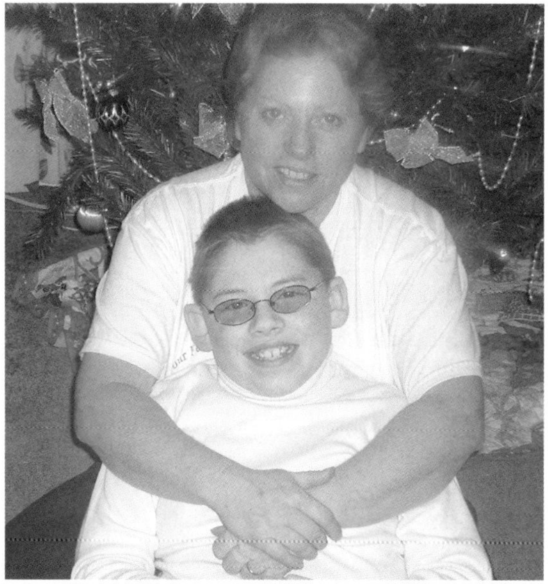

Andrew age 11

Contact:
hinkle1963@yahoo.com
828-862-3656

Andrew was diagnosed at 7 years

Biggest Challenge(s)

My biggest challenge has been getting the school system to have teachers better educated on what autism is and how to teach our children. And having them set up special programs to help my son excel in his own time. Other challenges have been: my own fears of having to raise and understand my child; learning how to help him to be his own person without trying to make him into something he is not.

Hearing for the first time that my child was autistic was the hardest for me and my family, until we learned more about autism. Learning how to deal with problems as they arise without becoming frustrated and angry.

Greatest Blessings

That God chose me to have this very special child to raise and love. How Andrew loves me back and challenges me to want to know him even more everyday. How my Church family, my family and friends have accepted him for who he is – a very loving special young man. How music brings out the best in his heart and mind. How it makes him shine above everyone else. How he brightens my day with his smile and love. Having friends who are willing to work with him and help teach music to him without payment, except to be able to be around him and enjoy his friendship. Having friends and family pray for him when he is having difficulties at school. Having Andrew as my son and friend.

Words of Wisdom

No matter what, you never give up on your child. Find his/her special talent and bring that forward and watch your child shine. Learn all you can to help your child. Stay on top of their education and health and not depend on the schools to know how to help them. Learn what is available to help them. Don't ever be afraid to ask questions about your child and their diagnosis.

Favorite Resources:

1) Teacch is an excellent source for help and learning more about autism.
2) www.autisum.org
3) Your local Library has excellent books.
4) www.autismresearchinstitute.com
5) *Treating Autism* by Stephen M. Edelson. Phd

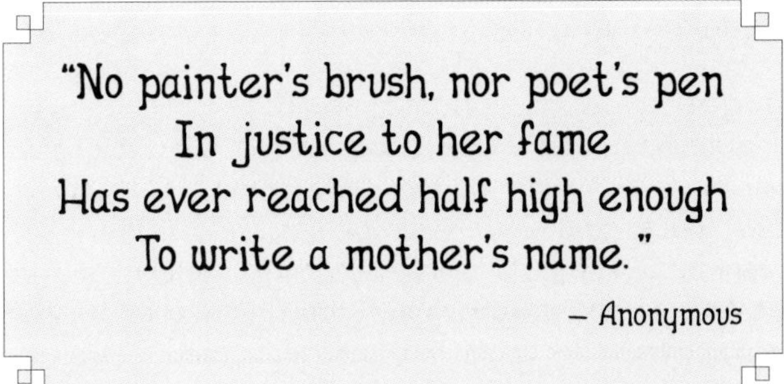

Bobbie & Vance

Kansas

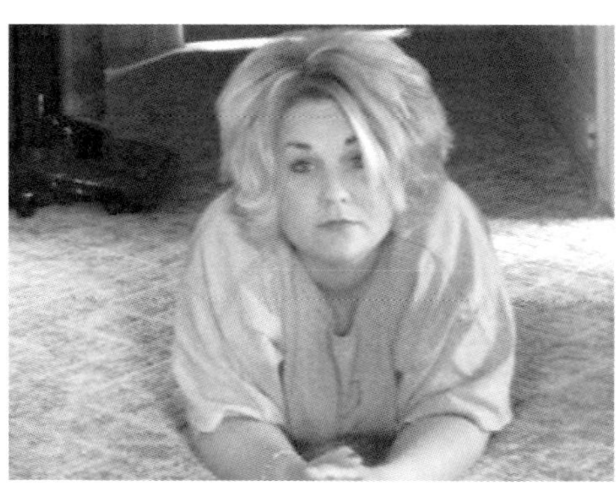

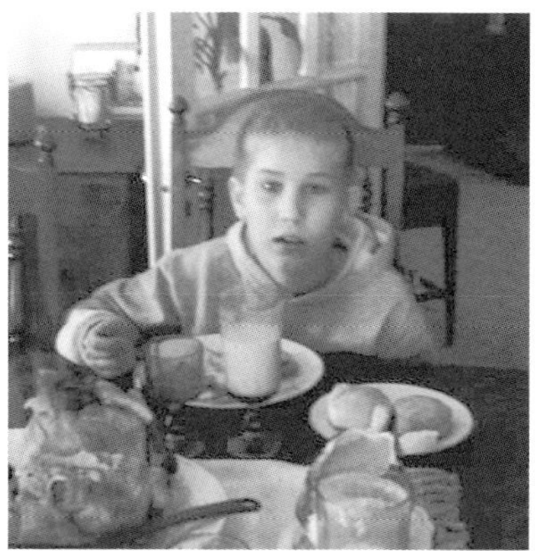

CONTACT:
aasfsg@sbcglobal.net

Vance was diagnosed at 10 years

BIGGEST CHALLENGE(S)

My son was diagnosed with Asperger's Syndrome at the age of ten and the biggest challenge we face is the lack of empathy to his situation. Often, common trips into the community prove to be heart-wrenching. People often do not understand why he has difficulty when reacting to the ultraviolet lighting in the stores, or when his stress level increases, he exhibits tics. I would like to yell at the top of my lungs to strangers and say, "Look past what you feel is 'weird' and just look at that young, beautiful face that is looking at you, because he doesn't understand why you scorn him, and just accept him for who he is!" Why do they feel the need to judge him, or me, as a parent? He's my son with the big beautiful, blue eyes that can tell you anything you would ever want to know about frogs, video games and the solar system. His vast knowledge never ceases to amaze me and while I'm aware of his talents and know how terrific he is, others do not, nor want to, at times. I have learned so much from my child, and while I know that we face daily tribulations, I also know that we will get through it.

Greatest Blessings

I would have to say being Vance's Mom is my greatest blessing. I truly am blessed to have this child a part of my life; it has taught me to look out beyond myself, my needs, and my desires and to truly see the world through his eyes. The things that I once took for granted, I now appreciate and take the time to relish in them. It still breaks my heart to have him come home in tears because he's experienced a problem at school due to his lack of being able to understand body language and facial expressions, or when someone finds it humorous to tell him a joke and he doesn't understand it, but comes home and asks me to explain it to him. It's moments like those and him telling me, "Mom, I love you and thanks for being my Mom". It's the little things like this that make me thankful for the blessings that have been bestowed upon me. I truly believe that I have been given this child to make me a better person and to educate and advocate for those that do not understand.

Words of Wisdom

I'm not sure what to really say here, except take time out for you. You are no good to yourself or your child when you are burnt out. I have found that taking too much on at one time, whether it be trying to be the Mom who participates in everything at school, from baking cookies, to participating in the PTO, as well as being an advocate for your child and other children like him, and working a full-time job can be rather overwhelming. It's OK to say "no." Have fun with your child! Turn the stereo on and dance around and be silly. Who cares if you don't have rhythm! Laugh often, hug often; it's the little things in life that really matter.

> "Laugh often, hug often:
> it's the little things in life
> that really matter."

Bonnie & Craig

Wyoming

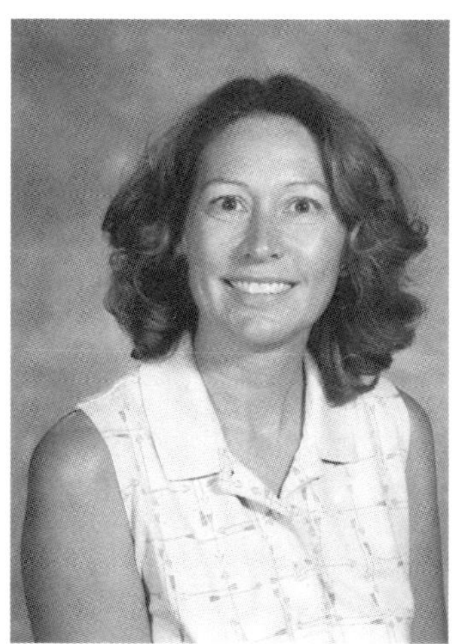

CONTACT:
geobw@trib.com

Craig was diagnosed at age 10

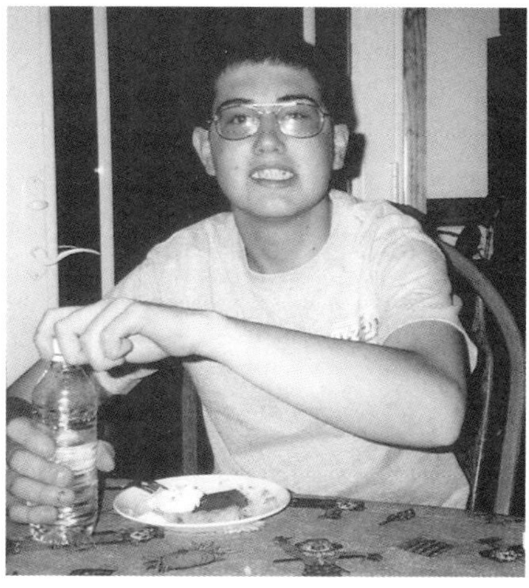

Craig November 2004

BIGGEST CHALLENGE(S)

My son was actually diagnosed about six years ago with autism, before that we had several different diagnostic "labels". They served a purpose. He got the services he needed and we can all be thankful for that. I am Bonnie, better known as "Craig's mom." Craig is diagnosed as PDD-NOS atypical autism. He is also ADHD and OCD. Craig is sixteen years old. He is fairly high functioning and ***very*** verbal. You know what I mean. His diagnosis includes a medically autistic caveat. Craig developed meningitis at the age of six months. He spent eleven days in the hospital, two of them comatose. After he recovered we knew we would have some challenges but we had no idea what to expect. As he has grown up we have just met each "challenge" as it came along. We developed a "bag of tricks" to intervene with his behaviors. We've also been lucky. We obtained early intervention services from a developmental child care center and later Craig transitioned into their preschool. From the preschool he moved into the public school system. We have been blessed with excellent staff and paraprofessionals. We have also been able to attend trainings and conferences that were beneficial to us along the way. In general all of the transitions have gone well.

Having always known that Craig would have special needs I don't know if I can present a greatest challenge although most recently we have been faced with a serious incidence of aggressive behavior. It has become so violent that we have sought out an alternative placement for academics and residence. We will hopefully find some resolution so he can return home, as we know he will someday. It is a perpetual roller coaster, but this will pass and keeping a positive attitude and a never give-up lifestyle will see us through. I believe that we have raised our children in a family environment that is nurturing and loving. We have never treated Craig any differently than our other children, although he does receive the special services that he needs.

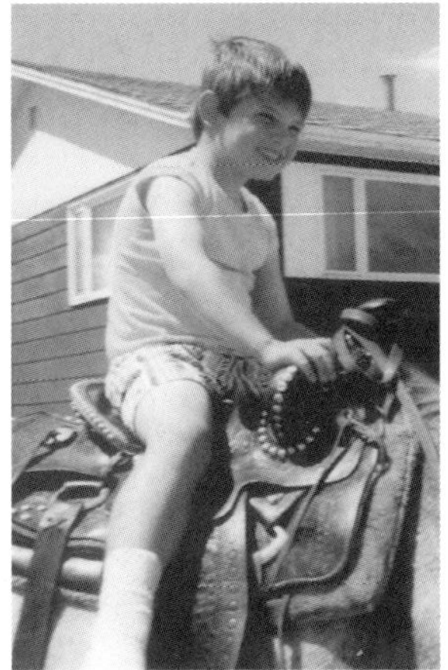

Craig 1994

Greatest Blessings

One of the blessings from Craig is his sense of humor. He can tell a joke, take a joke and he just "gets it" when something is funny. He also can get the giggles which we all know is an autistic trait, but it still can be appropriate. I guess the challenge is truly being given an opportunity to raise this young man and help him grow into a functioning individual in our community.

Words of Wisdom

I suppose the number one thing I would share with all of you is to take care of yourselves—everyday. You are the one best advocate for your child and it requires a lot of stamina. You must always be involved in **every** aspect of your child's life; home, school, work.

Make time for yourself everyday, (my 5:00 AM schedule may not work for you) and when necessary seek out some help. Child care providers are a great resource and as your child grows peers can be good advocates. There are agencies out there that provide respite care. Be honest. If someone offers to help, let them, and tell them what you need. Be happy, be thankful for each day. You can't go back, but you get a chance to do it again. Try again and share in the experience of living each day with your child.

Favorite Resources:

1) Future Horizons Inc., Arlington, TX
   They have a web site: www.FutureHorizons-autism.com
2) I also frequently check out the FDA web site and the drug manufacturers web sites for up-to-date information on medications.
3) *Social Skills Training* by Jed E. Baker, Ph.D.
4) *Asperger's... What Does It Mean To Me?* by Catherine Faherty
5) Parent Information Center, Buffalo, Wyoming
6) Parent Resource Center, Casper, Wyoming

Brenda, Andy, Jason & Jamie

Nevada

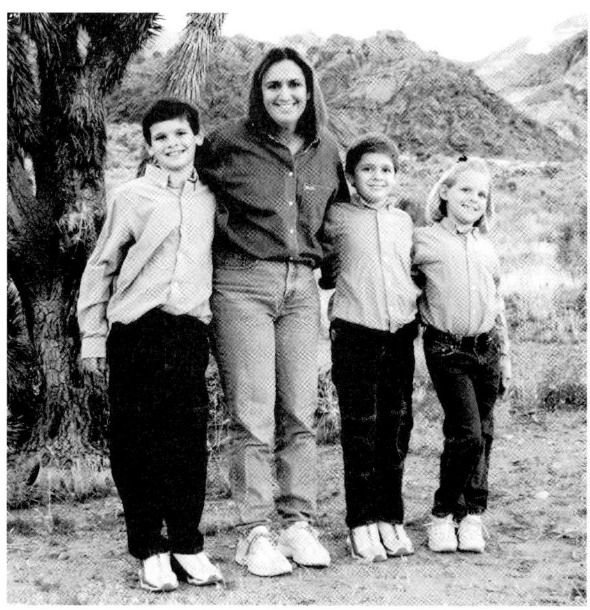

CONTACT:
702-249-KIDS
synergyhealer@yahoo.com
www.weseethelight.com

BIGGEST CHALLENGE(S)

1) Emotional – From an emotional standpoint, getting the news that your child has developmental delays, special needs, Autism, Aspergers Syndrome, Bipolar Disorder, or any seemingly chronic medical condition could be equated to facing death. For me it was. I came to understand through professional counseling and from Clinical Psychologist, Dr. Ken Moses, whose seminars on "The Normal Steps Experienced during the Grieving Process and Profound Loss", that I was actually experiencing a death. The 'death' I endured was that of a dream of healthy children along with the 'death' of my vision of a happy, 'normal', healthy family. Although my children are now basically healthy and gifted, I initially encountered shock facing the overwhelming reality of my situation with 2 boys, Andy (age 3) and Jason (age 1), both being placed on the Autistic Spectrum. My sadness deepened as my bright, socially perceptive daughter Jamie (age 5), exhibited behavior that indicated she was troubled by the stress in the house. With the help of Dr. Daniel Amen's book, *Change Your Brain, Change Your Life*, we used "Brain SPECT Scans" to understand how to address these issues. In time I came to the realization that only unstoppable persistence, inner strength, unconditional love, an undying quest for knowledge, insurmountable patience, and outside support including a synergy of the best medical care in the world could potentially heal these seemly overwhelming issues with which my children and I were confronted. We've had so much help, but most importantly, advice from our pediatrician, who pro actively alerted me to begin my boy's care within the first years of life, and a pediatric neurologist who has directed my children's care since age 2.

2) Physical – Over the course of 10 years the physical challenges I face include constant lifting, intense sleep deprivation (due to night time wake-ups from chronic seizure disorders, croup attacks, asthma and allergy attacks), and assisting my kids with basic needs due to global developmental delays. Obviously the day-to-day strain confronted by parents of children with special needs, especially moms of Autistic kids, can be very draining! Lifting and carrying kids is simply part of everyday life from early on due to developmental delays that prevent small children from crawling, walking, running, climbing or playing safely or age appropriately for many years or maybe ever. Constant vigilance is critical to insure the safety of the child and anyone else with whom there is contact.

3) Spiritual – *When Bad Thing Happen to Good People* by Harold Kushner is one of my favorite books that summarizes for me the challenges to my thought process that occurred as I faced the concept of 'Autism' with my family. Why did this terrible disability strike my children? Why me? What did my kids ever do to deserve this? Why couldn't they just been born healthy 'regular' kids? Why am I here on earth at all? Can I make it through, not just taking care of one child with 'special needs', but two or three? Do I have the strength to do this job as a single mom? Why don't people understand what I'm going through? How can I show people a way to treat my kids with respect? Will my kids ever say, "I Love You, Mom"? Will my kids always be in diapers? Will I ever have a life of my own again? Will they ever have independence…write their name, speak in full sentences, ride a bike, make friends, drive a car, go to college, live on their own, feel self confidence and the freedom of knowing they are productive, capable members of society? These spiritual questions have continued to run through my mind for years while raising my beautiful, compassionate, talented, loving, gifted, "special needs" kids on my own full-time as a single mom!

Greatest Blessings

1) Persistence –This overwhelming and terrifying process of fighting for my children's health has required constant optimism and perseverance, best summed up in Lynn Graghorn's book, *Excuse Me Your Life is Waiting*! I have purchased scores of copies for family and friends, and highly recommend it! One of my lifelong best friends, Amy (who coincidentally has a daughter, Rachel, with special needs) always tells me, "That which doesn't kill you makes you stronger!" Facing the complex and extensive issues surrounding neurological, psychiatric and other medical issues has taught me that incredible strength can be obtained through overcoming adversity against tough odds. My father, Dr. Robert Kravets, Psychiatrist for over 30 years, coaches me with his 'pep talks' using the "Power of Positive Thinking" and P.M.A. (Positive Mental Attitude) to inspire insurmountable hope and optimism into me and my children for the brightest future possible. My mom, Fern Kravets, teacher, Special Ed expert, and Guidance Counselor for over 30 years instills in me the values

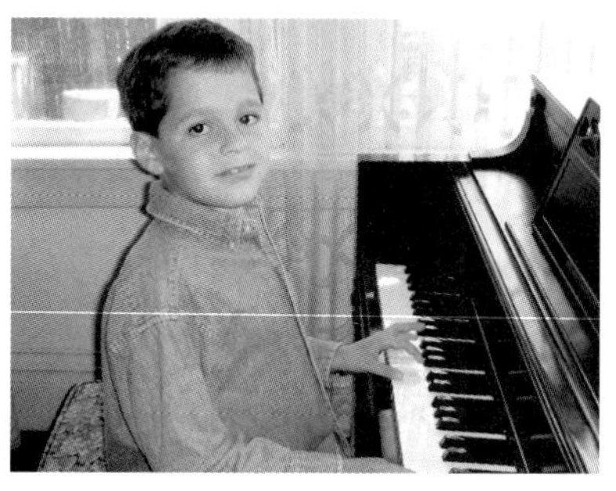

Jason age 8

of complete integrity and a tremendously consistent work ethic. My sisters Lisa and Aimee, and brothers, Howard, Mike and Steve, along with many extended family members, friends, neighbors and community members offer constant support, encouragement and love all along the path of my family's journey for a cure. My beloved Grandmother, Esther (age 87) is a constant source of light with her wealth of knowledge, articles and resources for furthering our learning on all subjects related to our family's healing and helping others in need.

2) Perspective – As Oprah, one of my greatest mentors has taught me, "What I Know For Sure" is children and generally all people suffering from special needs or any stressful issues or situations in their lives can provide a unique perspective to others not having to deal with these problems on a daily basis. I have developed incredible *insight* into what I am on earth to do with my life, immense *gratitude* for simply being alive to share my experience, strength and hope with others, *appreciation* for the unconditional love that surrounds me, *happiness* in the simple abundance I enjoy, *joy* in the precious gifts of lifelong honest friendships, *thankfulness* for my wonderfully loyal family, tremendous *compassion* and *empathy* toward others, *wealth of knowledge* on many subjects, *gifts of miraculous children*, *hope* for a bright future, and so much *ability to help others* in need from my personal experience of walking in so many shoes.

3) Unconditional Love – For optimal healing I have found it critical to maintain the ability to be a nonjudgmental, consistently unconditionally loving, totally accepting person. My special, gifted kids have the ability to share themselves completely openly, honestly, freely, and lovingly without the "normal" barriers of being self-conscious or insecure. Hugs, holding, frequent baths, splashing and simply allowing space to 'run free' have been crucial for them.

Words of Wisdom

A – Autism, Aspergers Syndrome, ADHD, Bipolar Disorder, Depression, OCD, ODD, Schizophrenia, LKS, seizure disorders and other related neurological and psychiatric disorders are all treatable, healable and may even be curable with the persistent pursuit of knowledge, unending patience, chronic unconditional unyielding love, and the creation of a synergy of positive influences, as Laura Day writes in her inspiring book, The Circle.

U – Ultimately OPEN-MINDEDNESS is the key to finding the right combination of therapies, vitamins, diet, exercise, medications, doctors, teachers, positive people (while eliminating negative people), friends, family and activities to enhance growth. For me keeping an open mind has also proved important in terms of maintaining a good relationship with their father Mike, who is with them whenever possible, and adds both emotional and financial support to their lives.

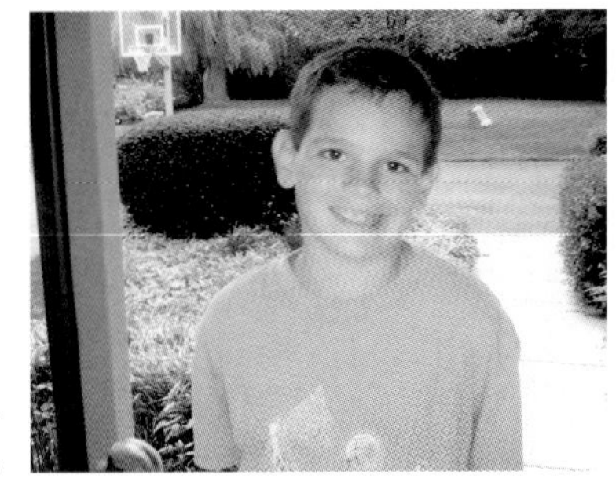
Andrew age 10

T – Together we can to what we could never do alone! By joining support groups, working through our schools systems and communities, and communicating constantly via phone, fax, voice mail, internet, web sights, books, and seminars, we can keep the flow of information going between and among our special needs communities and our medical research staff, who are working 24 hours a day in hundreds of countries worldwide to help improve the lives of our children everyday. Our goals are the same! SYNERGY WILL EXPEDITE THE PROCESS!!! SYNERGY means 1+1 = 3. Working together for the same goal will allow for better results to be accomplished more efficiently, faster and optimally for all involved. I have personally created a new non-profit organization called "WE SEE THE LIGHT". Its sole mission is to educate the world as a "National Teaching/Healing Institution for Special Needs Kids and Their Families & Synergy of Emerging Leaders for Global Health Care Management".

I – I need time to myself! Taking breaks from Autism or any issues that affect the family with special needs is extremely important. For the main caretaker to maintain good health and sanity, plans with friends, going to dinner and a movie, spa time, working out, reading a book, taking weekend vacations, and even finding a good therapist, can make all the difference in providing the entire family with a happy, loving, stable environment much of the time.

S – Self-Esteem is critical to the growth and development of any child, but especially important to a kid who begins life with disadvantages. Finding any hobby, interest, educational achievement, physical accomplishment or spiritual development should always be nurtured, totally encouraged, and rewarded -- no matter how small or seemingly insignificant. Each positive stepping stone leads a child down the road for future self-esteem on which to build a foundation of a healthy and more "normal" future. With even one simple skill a person can gain the feeling of accomplishment, paving the way to happiness in any other aspect of life.

M – Mom's generally in our society bare the burden of caring for the kids with special needs and adult children with disabilities today. As a single mom the most important advice I can give to others is to learn from the 'voices of experience' from famous world leaders and thinkers, and try to emulate them on a daily basis. I live my life with my children by spending as much 'quality time' or one-on-one time with them as possible, keeping in mind that the world does not and may never accept nor understand them the way that I do. Our family tries to live by example for optimal healing of mind, body, and spirit with integrity, hard work, balance, lots of laughter, multi-tasking, constant continuing education, proper diet, exercise, fresh air, vitamins, the minimal amount of medication necessary as prescribed by doctors, a synergy of positive influences, appreciation for nature, time together for games, the arts, and music, prayer, meditation, and lots of water for drinking, bathing and swimming!

Cara & Alex

Ohio

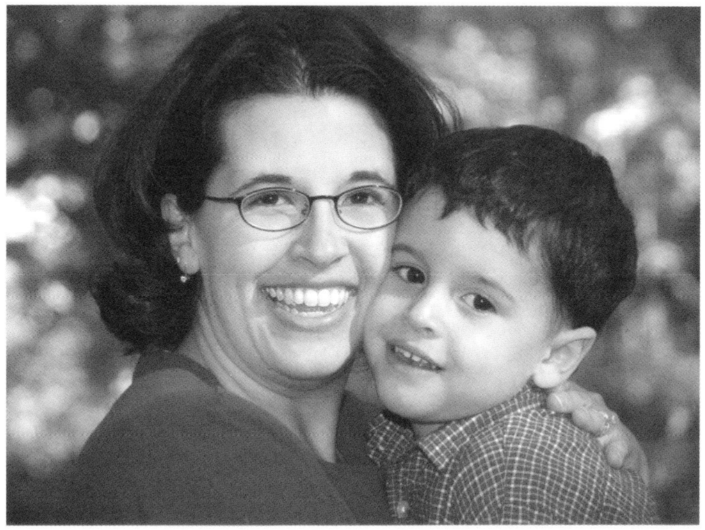
photos by Elizabeth Swansen

CONTACT:
korey_cara@msn.com

Alex was diagnosed at 3½ years

BIGGEST CHALLENGE(S)

Our biggest challenge at first was realizing Alex was autistic. Our general pediatrician at the time didn't think there was anything wrong with Alex. Since Alex was our first child and we didn't know much about autism, we were relying on him for that information. He gave us the "just wait and see" and "he's not in the corner rocking so he isn't autistic" statements! Once we got past that challenge, the everyday challenges with Alex were put into better perspective.

Since we now know he is autistic and have researched what that means, we feel we are better equipped to handle the everyday challenges. The current challenges are behavior problems at home, potty training, finding private services/getting services from the school and most importantly, paying for private services for Alex. The financial burden wouldn't be as much of a challenge if our medical insurance carrier would cover treatments for autism!!

Greatest Blessings

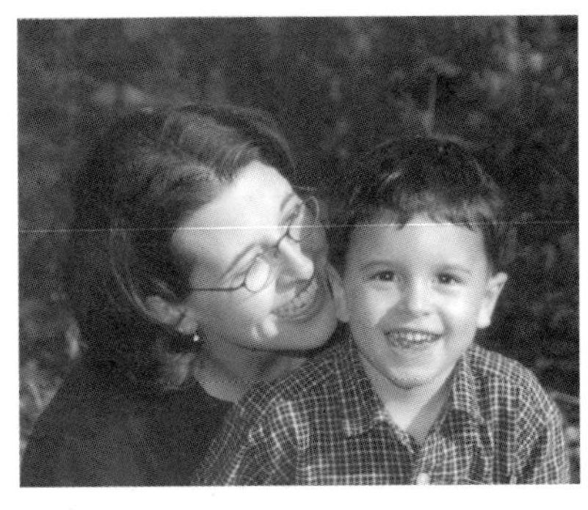

My greatest blessing is just having Alex in my life. Every little milestone seems even sweeter when you have a child with autism. He is so loving towards me that it melts my heart, especially since I know there are mothers of more severely autistic children out there that don't get to experience it. The second greatest blessing would be the support I have received from my husband. I feel that we have grown closer throughout all of this and will continue to grow closer as we raise Alex. I am truly blessed to have him as my husband. The third greatest blessing would have to be my best friend, Lisa. She was the one who told us that there was something wrong with Alex. I know that this was a very difficult thing for her to do. At first I was mad at her but I always knew deep down that she did it because she loves Alex like her own son. What a blessing she is.

Words of Wisdom

My most important word of advice is pray. I wasn't very good at praying before we found out Alex was autistic. I have found that, through prayer, I am able to get over the hurt that I first felt when we received the diagnosis. Through prayer, I have begun to understand the true blessing Alex is and will continue to be in my life and, more importantly, the direction God has for my life as his mother. It is an awesome thing to know that God has chosen me for this purpose here on earth.

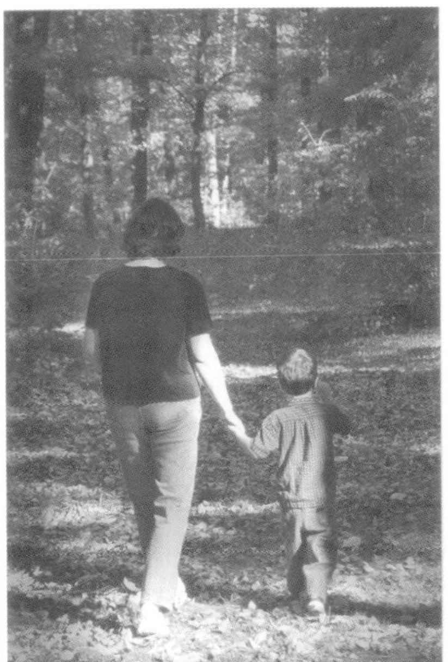

Secondly, read. You must research about autism. There is so much out there that it can be overwhelming. I know that I would prefer to be reading a good novel right now but find myself fascinated by stories of those who have had personal experiences with autism, particularly when written by someone who has autism. They are truly inspirational.

Last, but certainly not least, surround yourself with a good support group. This includes a good church home, friends, family, therapists, advocates, counselors, doctors, teachers, etc. You can't do this alone. God will provide a way through the help of those around you.

Carol & Nicholas

Missouri

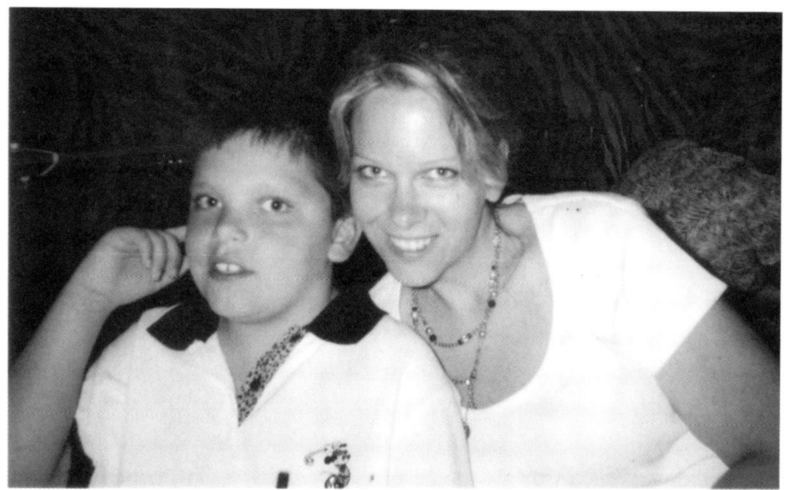

Nicholas age 7

Nicholas was diagnosed at 2 years

"Let parents bequeath to their children not riches, but the spirit of reverence."

– Plato

My Dream

by Carol Woehrle

I dream of the day you will be able
to tell me with your words
where it hurts, when you are sick.

I dream of the day you stand
at the end of the driveway
waiting for the school bus with your sister.

I dream of the day you graduate high school, as I shout,
"THAT'S MY BOY!" while they call your name
and you walk across the stage.

I even dream of the day you come home
and tell me you've fallen in love
and are marrying the girl of your dreams.
And if these dreams are not meant to be,
my dear son,
then I dream of the day I greet you in heaven
and meet my son - complete and whole
and perfect for the first time.

You will never disappoint me, my son,
even if these dreams don't come true.
For your value to me is not in these dreams,
but in the blessing of having known and loved YOU.

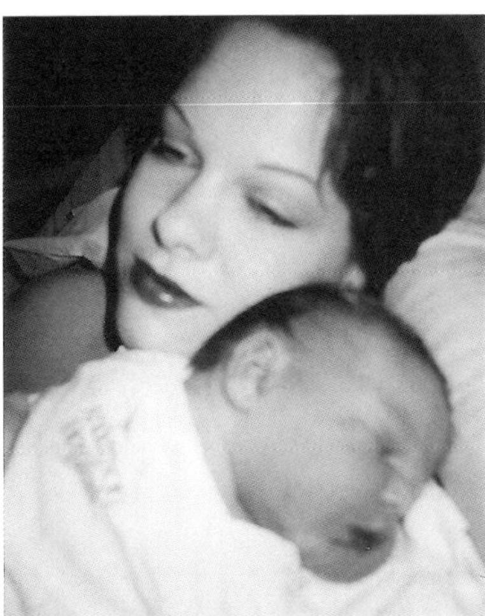

Written on the day
he was born
February 5th, 2000

Carol & Nicholas

Carolyn & Jacob

Arizona

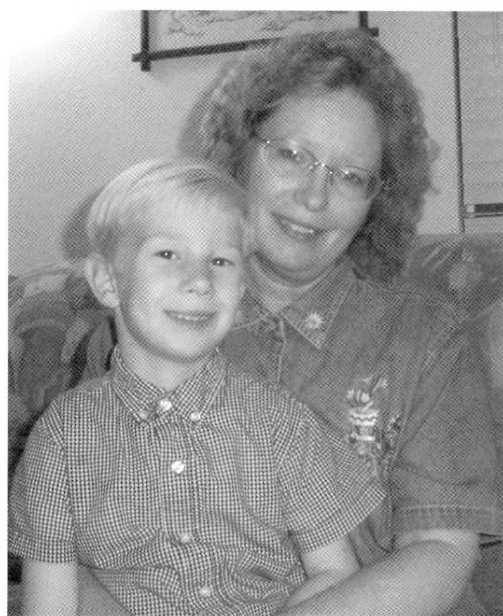

Jacob was diagnosed at 5 years

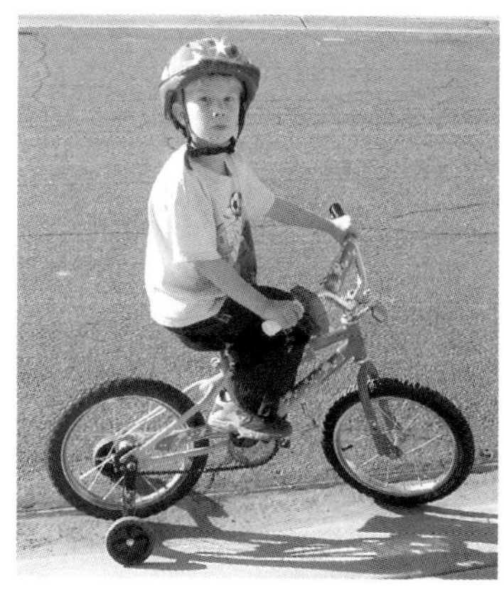

CONTACT:
623-412-3832
Montello1@juno.com

BIGGEST CHALLENGE(S)

My biggest challenge is that it has been so very difficult to communicate with Jacob; his inability to respond to my communication and the lack of feedback. Not knowing what he is feeling and his inability to tell me his feelings, I find I am in a constant struggle to find out his wants and needs.

I have two older sons who successfully met each milestone that came along. With Jacob it has been so extremely different. I just took the assumption daily that he would learn like my other boys, but that it would just take him a little longer. It has been hard trying to balance the fact that I have two typical sons and my youngest son is autistic. I am constantly trying to get as much help as I can for Jacob, while still trying to balance the needs of the rest of my family.

I went through all the childhood phases with my other two and when my third child arrived it was heart-wrenching to see that he was not meeting the same milestones and wasn't on the same time schedule of typical milestones. I have found that I make a lot of hopeful assumptions about Jacob. At times he gives me so little to go on that I project my own likes, dislikes and abilities onto him. I'm in a position where I'm guessing most of the time. I have to keep on guessing and trying to get through to him to the best of my ability. I don't believe I always achieve this but I know if I keep trying I cannot fail. To fail is to give up. My whole family has to help with this.

It can be difficult because we all have different ways of communicating. It involves more than just our words. It feels like a one-way communication sometimes as it is so exhausting trying to figure out if he understands.

It has been a lot of work to get help. I find myself constantly trying to educate myself, and people in general, about my son. Since his disability seems to be hidden at a first impression it is a constant challenge to go anywhere with him where there are new people and they don't know he has autism. I want him included and not excluded in the daily happenings of life.

As mothers we all experience some degree of stress when attempting to meet the care-giving demands presented by our children. It is hard to meet the demands associated with raising a child with a disability without some help. My husband and I can't do it all alone. Though it can be hard to ask for help.

Our family life revolves around Jacob, with interactions inside and outside the family being altered to accommodate his constant needs. I am often consumed with concerns for the physical welfare of my son, who would typically show no understanding of danger and couldn't even say his name if he got lost. I feel like I am always in a constant state of "high alert". It is hard to relax in his presence.

Greatest Blessings

One of my blessings came when I discovered intervention services for my son. When Jacob was 18 months I read an article in the *Arizona Republic* newspaper about evaluations and special education that I could call about. I discovered there was help available.

I cherish every accomplishment that he makes. Just to hear him learn to talk more and begin learning to ride a bike takes on an even bigger meaning for me especially since I have witnessed the joy of this with my older sons. I have found I don't take anything for granted and cherish every accomplishment that he makes, no matter how small.

Words of Wisdom

My words of wisdom are to try to seek as much help as possible and never give up. As his mother, I have found the most important thing I can do for my son is to be the best advocate that I can be. I encourage moms to continue to educate themselves and know their rights for education. As mothers we have to try and balance our lives – set apart time for ourselves, our husbands, our other children in the family; much like we do when we schedule doctor appointments and therapy appointments for our children.

I want to lead my son Jacob to the path of the best life possible for him. I have continued to see changes in him since birth and that has given me lots of hope. I can't look too far into the future because the doctors haven't been able to tell me what to expect for his future. Since it appears to be a mystery, with every child being created different, I have to take one step at a time. When I get really discouraged, wondering what kind of future he will have in his adulthood, I just keep reminding myself that he has made progress before my eyes from birth. I will always stay hopeful because God gave me Jacob as a special gift — my special blessing. I will continue to trust Him that He does have a special plan in life for Jacob.

Cate & Scott

Oregon

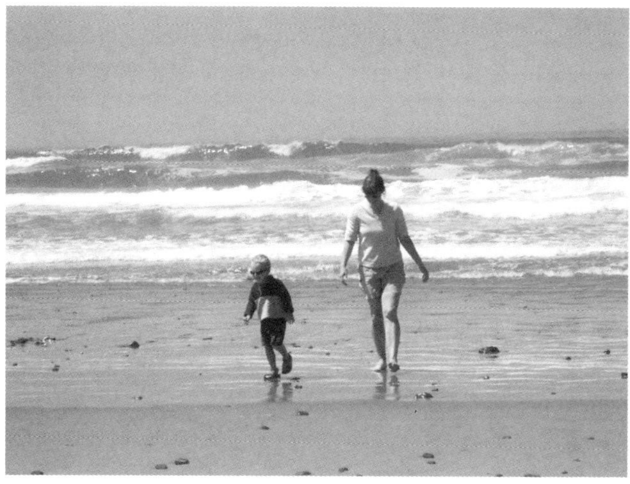

Scott was diagnosed at 3 years

Contact:
cate_hickman@comcast.net

Biggest Challenge(s)

There are many challenges about having a child with autism; it's overwhelming, scary, and isolating. The biggest one for me is always worrying about how life will be for him when he grows up. We are working hard to teach and prepare him, with the hope of "mainstreaming" him so he can live independently and have a good, happy life. Life is uncertain, but with autism (mercury-induced or otherwise), it is even more uncertain. Parents aren't around forever, and siblings need to have their own lives. I miss him so much, I wish he'd come back–I know he's trying. We were so close before he faded out (between age 2 to 2½, shortly after his brother's birth). This whole thing is still unbelievable and surreal. It's not supposed to happen.

Greatest Blessing

The greatest blessing through this is, and has been, our unwavering belief in him and his ability to learn and overcome obstacles and hopefully "be okay." Our ability to work very hard and constantly toward this goal is a blessing also. Finding others in our situation who understand helps a lot. I try to understand those who look at me blankly or don't want to deal with it and I think it comes from lack of understanding and fear. We've encountered some discrimination, but we can't let it get to us. We have to keep going and working hard for him.

Words of Wisdom

As far as words of wisdom, I'd suggest joining family support groups, like Families for Effective Autism Treatment (FEAT). This is too painful to go through alone. Thank goodness the Internet exists. When we found out what was going on almost two years ago, we searched for information and found a lot, fortunately. Like so many things, this is a world unto itself, something people never expect they'll be part of. Also a world we all want to escape, in hopes that our children will recover.

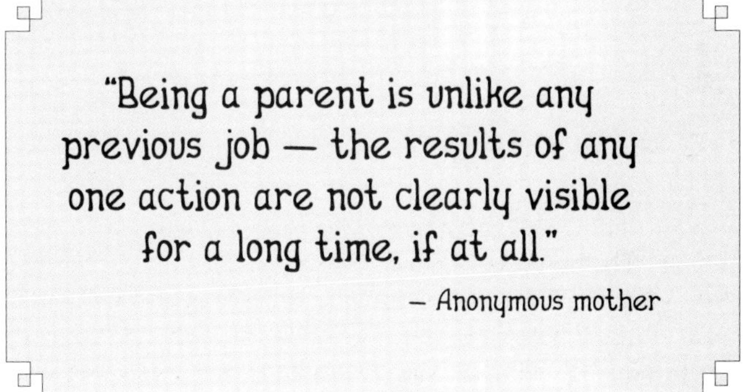

Christine, Cameron & Marcus

Indiana

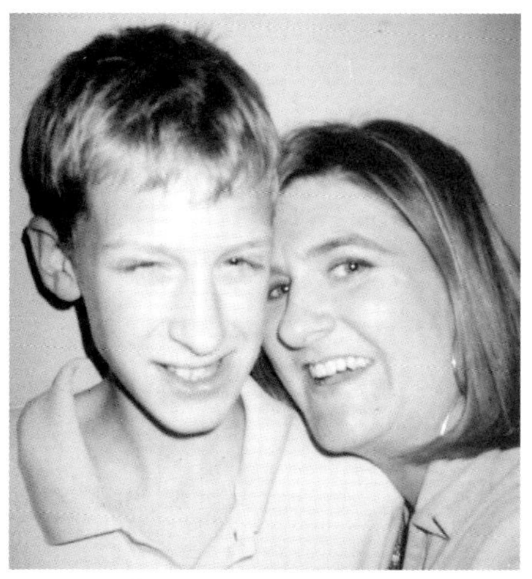

Christine and Cameron

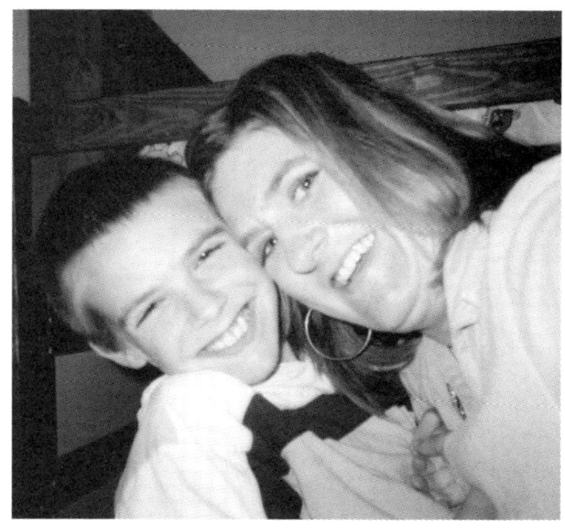

Christine and Marcus

CONTACT:
cmbheld@yahoo.com
Co-Founder, Co-President
www.AAIwalk.org

Cameron was diagnosed at 2 years old
Marcus was diagnosed at 17 months old

BIGGEST CHALLENGE(S)

My biggest challenge besides having three children, two with autism, is advocating for both my boys in their schools. Although, overall, our school district does well, I must still fight for things that I feel are necessary for their success. The hardest part for me is keeping my emotions in check and being calm and factual during a meeting. No one will listen to a crying, screaming, know-it-all mom, so learning the law and how to apply it has been a huge plus.

I have taken classes and seminars that will help me present a knowledgeable and law-based argument. It really works without drawing in lawyers and confrontation. One thing I have to remember is when I am done fighting for something with one of my sons, I must wipe the slate clean in order to challenge the same administrators for something else for my other son. Holding grudges will only make the process harder. Prayer and good support from other moms dealing with autism helps.

Greatest Blessings

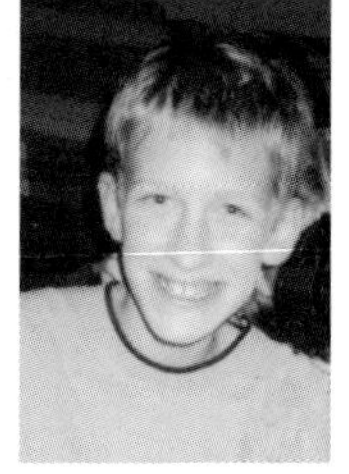
Cameron age 12

My greatest blessing is, by far, my children's honest, contagious laughter. Their giggles are delightful and have made many a scrooge snicker. Their smiles ar heart warming and wash away any stigma that autistic individuals are cold and emotionless. They have their difficulties, but they are happy children.

Another wonderful blessing is all the unique and astonishing moms I have met who deal with autism and work hard all day in and day out to make their children's lives as productive and well-adjusted as they can. What a joy and inspiration they have brought to my life. Thank you all, especially the parents in my AAI group. You are the best!

Words of Wisdom

Know your child!! Know his/her moods, likes, dislikes, habits, needs, and signals that trigger behaviors. Let him/her be the person they want to be and accept him/her for who they are, not who you want them to be or become. If he obsesses with maps, let him plaster his room with them! If he wants to recite a movie and dress-up as a character, let him. Enjoy their uniqueness, and embrace that they are different. They will be happier and you will be proud of who they really are.

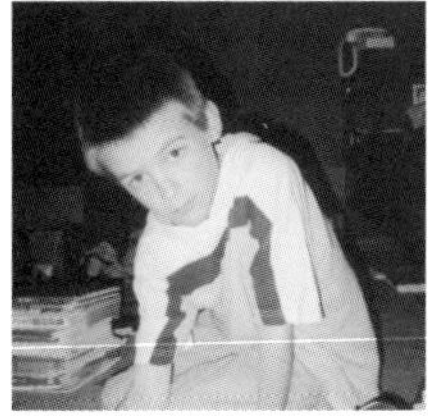
Marcus age 11

"Let him be the person
they want to be
and accept him
for who they are,
not who you want them
to be or become.
If he obsesses with maps,
let him plaster his room with them!"

Christine & Peter

Massachusetts

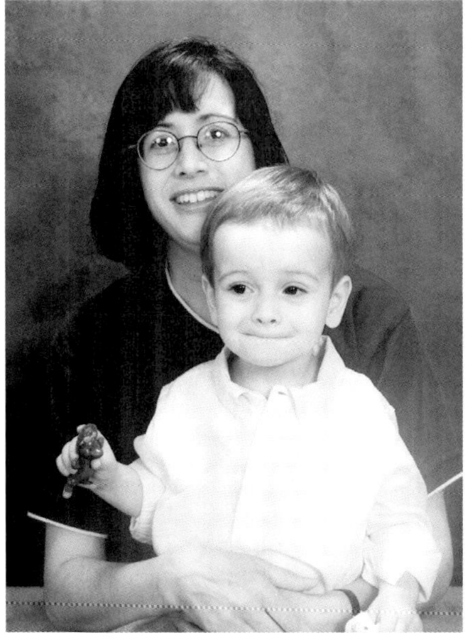

Peter age 3

Peter was diagnosed at 19 months old

CONTACT:
781-910-5222

BIGGEST CHALLENGE(S)

When Peter was born there was no denying he was perfect. Ten perfect fingers and toes. He relished everyone and everything. He loved Dougy, the little boy next door, the most. Our first born was more than we had hoped for in every way. We have had the joy of this child. He was our gift and we recognize this and cherish him in our hearts. I remember what his voice sounded like…and it is beautiful.

By eighteen months, he was so very different from the effervescent child we gave birth to. He had disappeared starting at fifteen months and was diagnosed at nineteen months. He no longer recognized the boy next door. This new child, in Peter's body, was so much needier, and determined to exclude us from his world. With little to no subtle social gestures, it became hard maintaining more than a moment of his attention.

The biggest challenge was putting one foot in front of the other while desperately hoping for our child to return. My boy sang, had an imagination, and it was obvious how everything in life had excited him. What happened to him? What stifled him? Could this have been avoided? This is life, not just ours, but many persons. Where are the answers?

Greatest Blessings

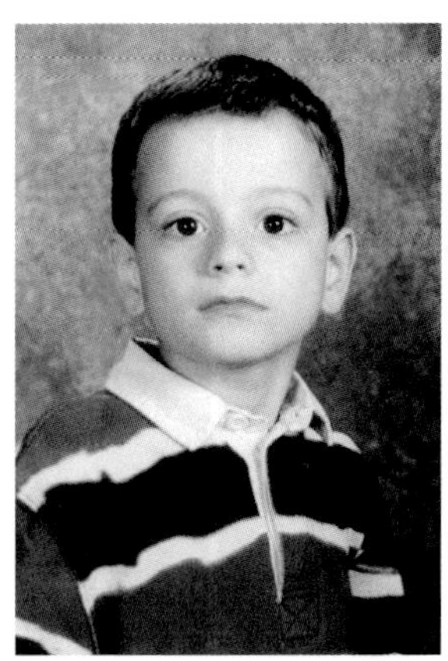

Often we are admired by loving people trying to understand what it is like to be in Peter's life daily. I am always stunned to hear this because everyday we wake up to Peter and his limits. He wasn't given an option and neither were we. We got through those first years, coping with all the unanswered questions… because of our love, inexhaustible love, and never wavering love. A love more overwhelmingly a part of us than any situation Peter's disorder could put us in. My husband and I are a team; our goals are clear, and we are united. We don't allow anyone to divide our attentions.

I have become a teacher, taking every opportunity to teach strangers, children, institutions (school districts, community service providers), maitre d's, security at airports, and my child, Peter, what is appropriate. Throughout this, I have acknowledged everyday angels who quietly come up and ask if I need assistance when my child has two handfuls of my hair in his hands, or who have let us slip past even though the child "looks normal" but really needs to go first. Peter is non-verbal, and we feel his frustration daily.

He is now eight, strong, tall and handsome. He has personality, a kind heart and love that catches our breath daily. He had regressed every year for four years after his first regression, but now has had a year of progress. Assessments tell me he is more like a two year old, which is definitely better than a nine month old. Hope is eternal.

Words of Wisdom

When this all started I cried each day. Then I realized this happened to Peter, my child, my baby, and not to me. I owed it to him to learn the early intervention ropes, the alternatives to treating his disorder and for enlightening all who work with him to demand and expect more from him. I am his Mother and take pride in every sign of progress, become bear-like when I feel he is threatened, and am thankful to be so fully a part of his life.

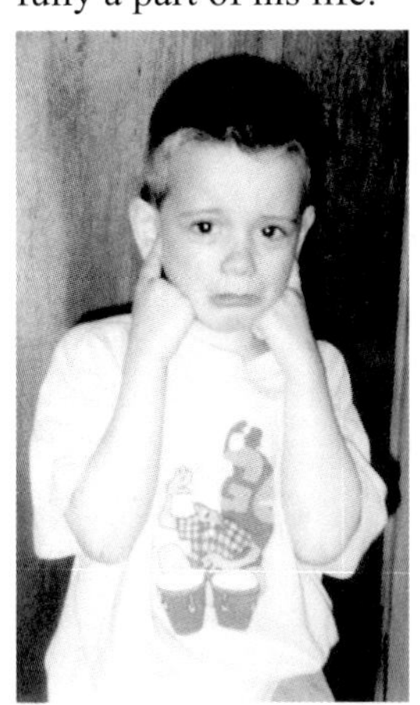

Looking back over the past six years, I realize that I now need to understand how Peter's condition has affected the lives of family and friends. It is time for me to help them get to know Peter. I am amazed at how many people have admitted to me that when he was younger, they thought I was making up problems. Now they admit it was good I was so bull-headed about his deficiencies. It is forgivable not to understand, not wanting to be involved; it is very forgivable when you realize that it is never too late to be more a part of his life now.

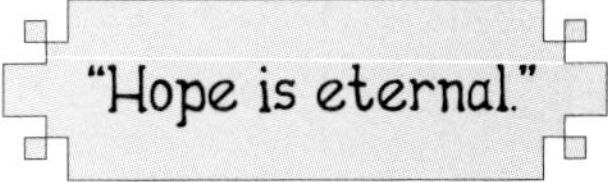

Christy & Terry

Colorado

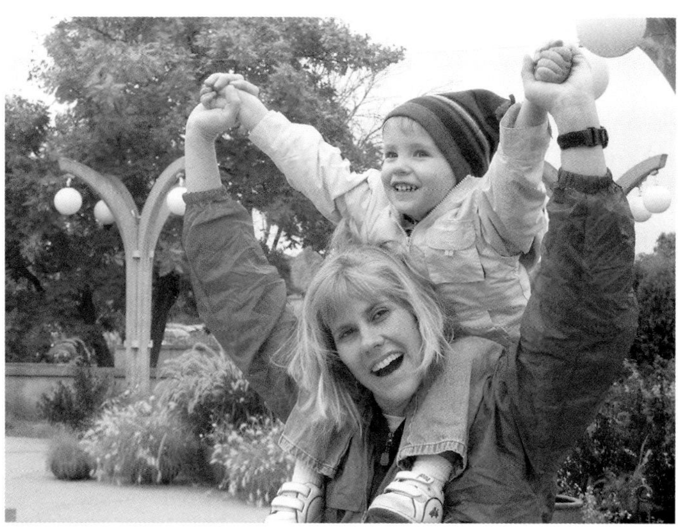

Terry was diagnosed at 2 years 3 months

CONTACT:

christyshoemaker@yahoo.com

BIGGEST CHALLENGE(S)

A nagging feeling that something just wasn't right:

Why is Terry the only one screaming when I put sunscreen on him at the park?
What are these stomachaches that keep him awake for hours at night?
Why won't he say "mama" and "dada" anymore?

Anxiously waiting to hear what our pediatrician said at Terry's two-year checkup:

"Don't worry. Boys develop language later.
I'd wait another 6 months before getting a speech evaluation."

Still feeling that now-familiar knot in my stomach:

What if he doesn't start talking? Will I ever hear his voice?
Will he ever want to play with sand, play-dough, or finger paint like other kids?

Disbelief from friends and family when we voiced our concerns:

"Kids develop at different times."
"His Uncle Ken didn't talk until he was 3. Even Einstein was a late talker."
"Naw, he's a smart kid."
"Don't worry so much."

Sharing the diagnosis and receiving what can only be described as sympathy cards:

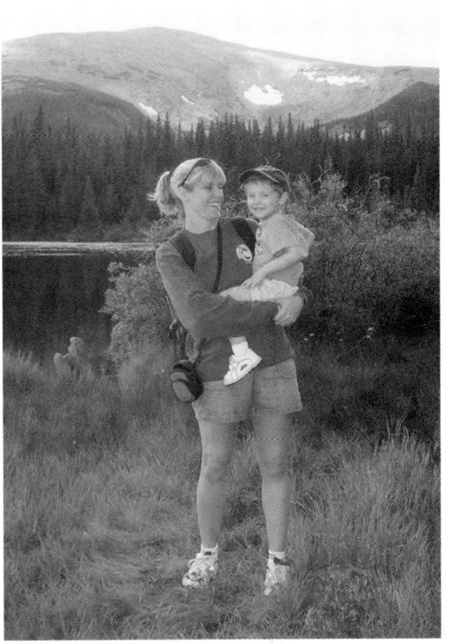

"He doesn't look autistic to me."
"You'd never know it."
"Autism is like ADHD used to be. Now everyone thinks they've got it."
"You don't want to get saddled with a label."

Fearing Sunday school, playgroups, and childcare where his symptoms might be misunderstood as misbehavior:

"I can't get that kid to come over and wash his hands. He won't listen to me!"
"Your son refuses to follow directions. Does he have ANY rules at home?"

Being thrown into the role of educator and advocate while still going through our own emotional processing of the diagnosis:

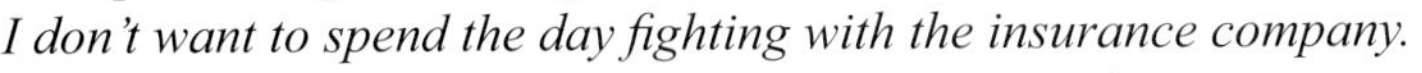

I don't want to spend the day fighting with the insurance company.
I don't want to have to know what our rights are before we meet with the school district.
I don't know what caused Terry's autism.
I don't know what will happen to him . . . to us.
I don't know what you can do to help.

Regular parenting challenges feel insurmountable:

How long will I have to take him to the bathroom every 20 minutes?
Will we ever be able to cut his hair when he is awake?
Will we always have to visit a new doctor's office ten times before our first appointment so it becomes familiar to him?
Will he ever sleep through the night?

Overwhelming responsibility and guilt:

Am I implementing enough of the right early intense interventions?
Was it a mistake to vaccinate according to our pediatrician's recommendations?
Should we have known we were passing on bad genes?

Struggling with trying to maintain a happy, balanced life for all of us:

Will I ever have a day when I don't feel guilty for not making it therapeutic enough?
Will we ever have the confidence to think about having another child?
Is it even possible to catch my breath and have time to focus on my goals and career?

Greatest Blessings

Loyal friends who bravely broke through my denial:

"I noticed Terry didn't really look at me when I asked him about his magnets."
"What did your pediatrician say about Terry's speech delay?"
"In my practice we suggest getting an evaluation right away."
"I would just want to be able to rule out anything serious. . . like autism."
"It couldn't hurt to check it out now instead of waiting. . . and it might really help."

Compassionate, knowledgeable professionals who have become part of Terry's team, part of our **family**:

Terry watches out the window when I tell him his OT, Kate is coming over.
This music class is perfect. No one bats an eye that Terry is too overwhelmed to participate.

Becoming so tuned in to Terry's development that we can look at the tiniest little step with great appreciation and pride:

If our child had been typical, would we have taken all this for granted?
Would we have celebrated his first bite of birthday cake, finally, at age 3?
Would we have cheered at his first request for finger paint?
Would hearing him say the words "bubbles" and "blow" bring tears to our eyes and hope to our hearts?

Finding child care workers and babysitters who may not have backgrounds in autism but whose caring and generous hearts responded with:

"So how can I help Terry?"
"How can we make this a happy, safe place for him?"
"I just love working with Terry, please don't stop coming here."

Friends and family who continue to welcome us into their lives when we feel a bit removed from the world:

"Tell us what we can do to support all three of you."
"Let's get our kids together again for a play date."
"Please bring Terry along!"

Working together with his father, my husband, to meet Terry's many needs:

Did he get much vestibular input today? He is just spinning around in circles.
Don't forget to give him his supplements after he eats.
Guess what? We went to the shoe store and Terry actually let the guy measure his foot!
I need a break. Can you take over for awhile?

Feeling blessed every single day to get to spend it as Terry's mom:

"Come Mom!" he says when he wants me to get the puzzle we do together.
"I want Mommy lay down," he says when he wants to snuggle or fall asleep.
"Mom!" he smiles and says when he sees me walk into his preschool classroom.
"Mom," he says in his sweet voice and I think, 'Wow. . . that's me.'

Words of Wisdom

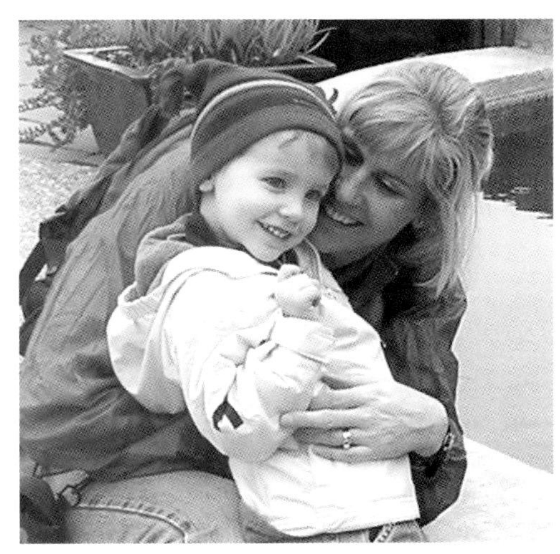

Accept the challenges:

It is work. It is crazy, busy, hard and emotional work to be a parent of autism. I am learning how to be the parent Terry needs me to be.

Find the blessings:

I have a tiny window into Terry's world. It is a window that is slowly growing larger. With every little success, we celebrate. With every new day we look for magic and joy together.

Hold onto hope:

Autism is a part of who Terry is and of the journey we are on. It is a package deal and I wouldn't trade it for anything.

Favorite Resources:

RDI Information:
Autism Asperger's: Solving the Relationship Puzzle by Steven E. Gutstein
Relationship Development Intervention with Young Children by Steven E. Gutstein and Rachelle K. Sheely http://www.connectionscenter.com/

Hanen Class Information:
More Than Words by Fern Sussman
http://www.hanen.org/

General Autism Information:
http://www.autism-society.org
http://www.orgsites.com/co/asbc/ (Local Chapter of the ASA)

"Accept the challenges.
Find the blessings.
Hold onto hope."

Cindy & Gavin

Wisconsin

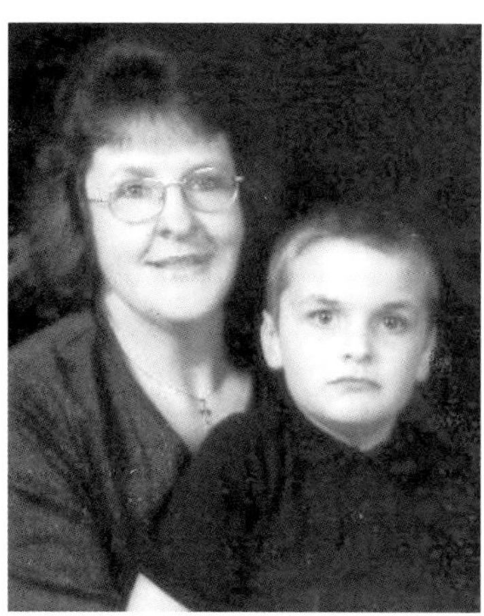

CONTACT:
heavenly_angels7@hotmail.com

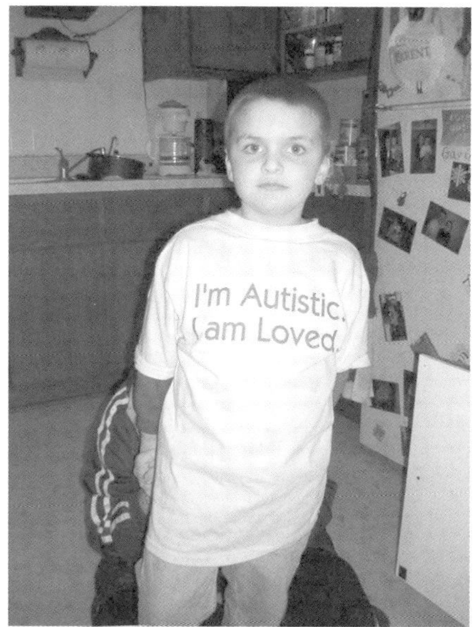

Gavin was diagnosed in June 2001

BIGGEST CHALLENGE(S)

One of my biggest challenges, being a mother with a special needs child, is doing everything humanly possible to make him better. These are children with various biological issues, and autism can be corrected with early intervention. There is hope, our kids can be restored. It takes time and a lot of patience. I do a lot of work with my son's diet. He has food allergies, so the Gluten Free, Casein Free, Yeast Free, Low Sugar diet has helped him. He has problems with yeast overgrowth, so we had to also do the Specific Carbohydrate Diet as well to heal his gut and intestinal tract. We have used many supplements to help this healing process. He will probably always have autism, which is fine, because we love him know matter what. However, I hope that in my lifetime I can heal him, with the help of others, to be the best that he can be. That is my goal.

Another challenge is the constant fight to obtain services for these children. In home Applied Behavior Analysis (ABA) has helped our child learn so many things. Every little step in learning is such a huge accomplishment to independence. There is such joy as a parent you feel in your heart when they have mastered a program and gained new skills. They need this treatment before school age so that they do not slip between the cracks of the system. Early intervention is the key to unlocking these children.

Greatest Blessings

Having a child with autism has sent into our life some amazingly, wonderful people. These individuals that work with our son truly care and love him. Their heart is in their work. It is more than just a job to them, they see the daily rewards of working with these kids. They are special people, who work with special kids. They have added so much to our life and helped our son a great deal. We are very grateful to all of them. Our provider, therapists, teachers, and doctors all have played a very important role in bringing Gavin to where he is today and where he will be in the future. Having Gavin has made our family realize how important good nutrition is for the body. We have all become more health conscious because of him. Having a large family to help out has made the burden on me as a mother not quite as hard. I am grateful for the help they give Gavin and I. We are not alone, God is guiding us through this journey. He never sends us more then what we can handle. Putting my trust in Him to get us through the uncertain times has helped us. Seeing our son achieve things we never thought possible always makes us realize there is a smart boy behind those big green eyes. He has come so far at such an early age, yet has so much further to go. Whatever the future holds for him I am sure he will do great things. We are extremely proud of him.

Words of Wisdom

We are all these children have. We have to remain strong voices for the voiceless. Be strong advocates for your children. Become part of a support group, if you do not have one in your area start one. I did! It helps to learn from others. It is our responsibility to make autism awareness known. If we don't who will? Try every avenue when it comes to helping your child. If one treatment or therapy does not work, try something different. They can learn, they can get better, you just have to figure out what works for your individual child. Autism is a spectrum, what works for one may not work for another. You can make a difference in the lives of children with autism. Parents who care and are willing to help are an e-mail away, feel free to contact me about any issue concerning autism spectrum disorder. Remember, make time for yourself. As mothers, we feel we can rule the world. We can do everything. Often times if we do not take a little time for ourselves the world can cave in. If we are not taking care of ourselves who will take care of our child with autism or our family. If we are not healthy and happy they will not be either. Joining a gym has really helped me manage stress in my life. I would recommend it to anyone. If you cannot take the time for that, just a walk outside or ride a bike. Get out, breathe the fresh air, enjoy the beauty around you. You and your family will be glad you did. God Bless You ALL.

Favorite Resources:

1) *Biological Treatments for Autism and PDD*, Dr.William Shaw, 2001
2) *Breaking the Vicious Cycle: Intestinal Health Through Diet,* Elaine Gottschall, 1994
3) *Children with Starving Brains,* Dr. Jaquelyn McCandless, 2003
4) *Facing Autism*, Lynn M. Hamilton, 2000
5) *Special Diets for Special Kids, One and Two* Lisa Lewis, 1998, 2001
6) *Unraveling the Mystery of Autism and PDD: A Mother's Story* , Karyn Seroussi, 2002
7) *What Your Doctor May Not Tell You About Children's Vaccinations,* Dr. Stephanie Cave

Damaris & Timothy

Australia

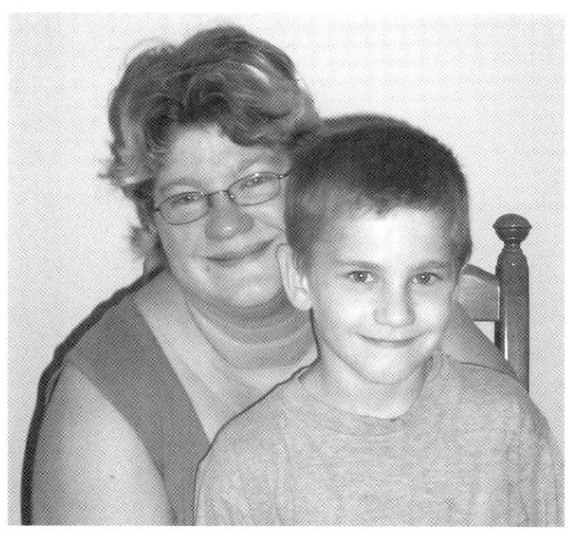

CONTACT:
damaris@optusnet.com.au

Timothy was diagnosed at nearly 7 years

BIGGEST CHALLENGE(S)

My beautiful boy's name is Timothy, and he is nearly 8 years old. He was first diagnosed with ADHD after my mother (on mother's day of all days) told me a few years ago that my child was no longer welcome at her house. I was told, through my husband, that we had no parenting skills and that we did not know how to discipline our child. That prompted me to pull my head out of the sand and recognize that, yes, my son was different than the others. After the ADHD diagnoses, along came severe eczema as well as Central Auditory Processing Disorder, meaning that he can't deal with background noise. Late last year he ran away from school hoping to find me at home so that I would listen to him; as teachers at school weren't listening as far as he was concerned. This prompted the school to allow his specialist, my husband, and I, to call for a conference meeting and Asperger's was diagnosed. At this meeting, as a lot of loop holes had been filled, he was then ascertained to receive the highest support you can in this state. He is now 2 out of 6 hours each school day in his normal classroom and the rest in the Special Education Unit. A lot of days he doesn't even make through that.

Parents and other students certainly don't know how to take my son. He so wants to play but it is like there is a force field stopping him. He knows that 7 year old boys have friends but he doesn't know why or what they are good for, and how to get them, let alone keep them. Facial recognition is something that we are really working on at the moment, as well as expressing his feelings instead of just exploding. Speech/Language has always been a problem as well.

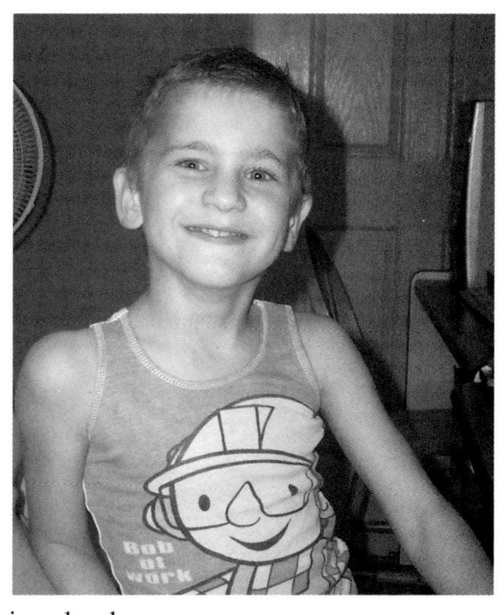

He is very misunderstood by the school concerning what can be expected of him. If he was left alone in a quiet area to do math, read or computers there would never be a problem. He loves those. No communication involved, you see.

Playtime, when he does do it, is always on his terms and he decides the rules just so that he knows what is going on and feels in control.

Greatest Blessings

I wish there was an out for Timothy, or a little pill that would make it all go away. But then I look at him asleep and think just how lucky I am that he is in my life. Without him I would not have learned to be more empathetic, tolerant and aware of others' point of view. I have been able to easily welcome others into my home and know that they feel comfortable as they know that I am being genuine. I know that he has a hard road ahead of him but with my husband and I, as well as the band of specialists that we have around us now, I know that we will get there in the end.

Words of Wisdom

It is all about early intervention. If you are not happy with the service you are getting from one specialist, go to another. I have gone through 4 pediatricians alone and 2 psychologists. And I am sure that I will have more changes to do yet as he grows older. Medication is also not right yet. His anxiety is extreme and tolerance levels are not high, but again we are working on it hour by hour.

"Patience and perseverance have a magical effect before which difficulties disappear and obstacles vanish."

– John Quincy Adams

Deborah & Devin

Alabama

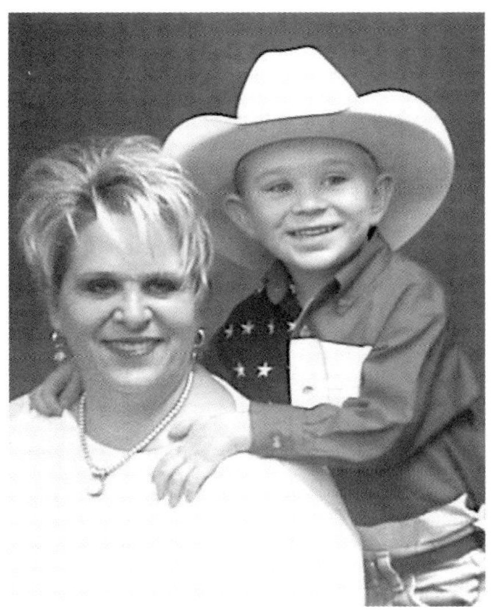

Devin is diagnosed with Aspergers

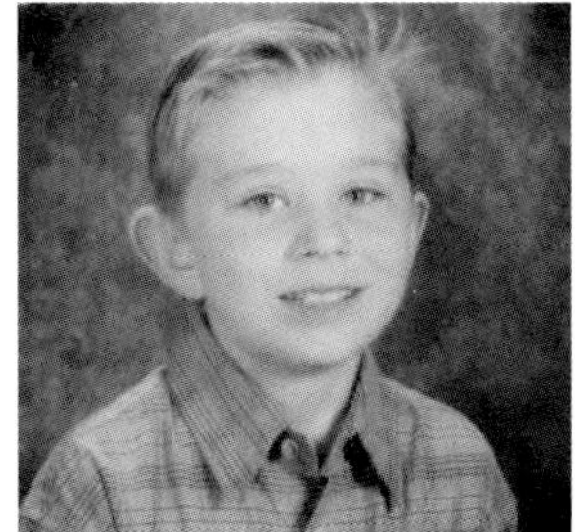

Devin at 7 years old

Devin was initially diagnosed as ADHD at 5 years of age. His kindergarten year had become a very troubled time in his life. Devin had lost his father and I thought that the death of his father, combined with various changes in his life (such as my remarriage and his learning that he was going to be a big brother), were surely the cause of Devin's behavior in his kindergarten class. That was a lot for a 5-year-old.

During this year, I wasn't concerned with him "staying in the lines while coloring". After all, the teacher kept telling me how smart he was. Besides, I thought, maybe it wasn't his "fine motor skills", maybe he just didn't care if his picture was pretty — maybe that was normal. However, during the course of the kindergarten year, Devin had a problem going to the bathroom and it became apparent that something just wasn't right. I took him to his regular pediatrician to rule out physical problems and to ask about possible treatment. The pediatrician was slightly familiar with ADHD and gave me information on the subject. I then took him to a psychologist and a counselor, if the problems were due to the death of his father, I felt that they would pick up on this and council him. I kept in mind that this was lot for a five year old to deal with. I also knew that the family changes—a step-dad, a new sister, were challenging. I wondered if all these things stressed him out.

The professionals tested him and gave him the diagnosis of ADHD, ODD. The psychiatrist had asked about Devin's history and I revealed all of the facts from his complicated birth to his biological father being diagnosed bi-polar. We went through a lot of different medications for his ADHD, but still I felt as if there were something else that I wasn't catching with Devin. In fact, things got so bad that Devin started to have thoughts of suicide. He'd say, "I can't do anything right, I just want to hurt myself, die"... "I'm so stupid". I became very disturbed by this and knew I wasn't dealing with just an ADHD problem. I was at my wits end. I was scared and in need of a different opinion. My heart ached for my son. I didn't know what to do. The psychiatrist was not much help. She prescribed medications for his ADHD and listened.

In the first grade, things became more complicated for Devin. Riding a bike was an issue. Tying his shoes became an issue. There were a lot of things that Devin should have been learning, but couldn't. Other people were quick to judge and place the blame on me for bad parenting. I felt horrible as a parent, but proved myself otherwise. We weren't sure if Devin wasn't interested in learning to tie his shoe or ride his bike, or simply just didn't want to. We eventually learned that Devin was only interested in certain things like play station, the computer, Pokemon, and Yu-Gi-Oh. This became a daily problem at home and at school. We set limits and goals for Devin. We felt we were trying creative ways to help him become interested in things that he had to be interested in, such as school.

Devin went through a series of tests at the school because of an IEP being established. We found that he was well above average after taking two different IQ tests. They could not believe his score and double checked themselves, making sure it was graded properly.

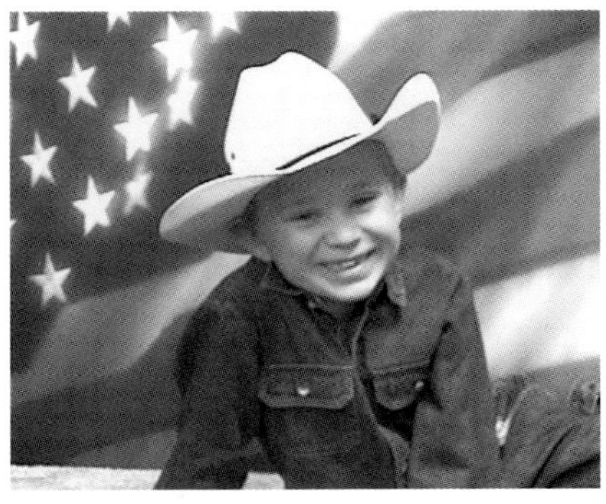

In second grade, a new counselor recognized the symptoms of Asperger's Syndrome and recommended we take him to an out-of-town doctor. Although Devin was diagnosed with Asperger's Syndrome, Language Disorder with High IQ; the school decided he didn't need any further help because he was doing so well. At a recent IEP meeting they doubted his diagnosis because he was doing well academically and socially. I felt like a real heel. I felt they were saying, "There is nothing wrong with him, so why do you insist on wanting it to be?" Nevertheless, at this IEP meeting we decided the school would pay for a second opinion. Sure enough, the second opinion came back: "diagnosis is correct." The people who tested Devin also had several suggestions for the school. Some of the suggestions they fear as they "are not the norm."

Sometimes I feel like I am the only parent in that school that pushes to get what's needed for my son. If it weren't for the IEP meetings, nothing would be accomplished, I still have to "fight" and push my way to get them to listen. I learn as I go. If it hadn't been for our new counselor, we wouldn't be at this point. I am not grateful that Devin has Asperger's Syndrome, but I am grateful we have the "correct diagnosis" so we know how to treat it.

Deborah &Devin

Deborah & Holly

North Carolina

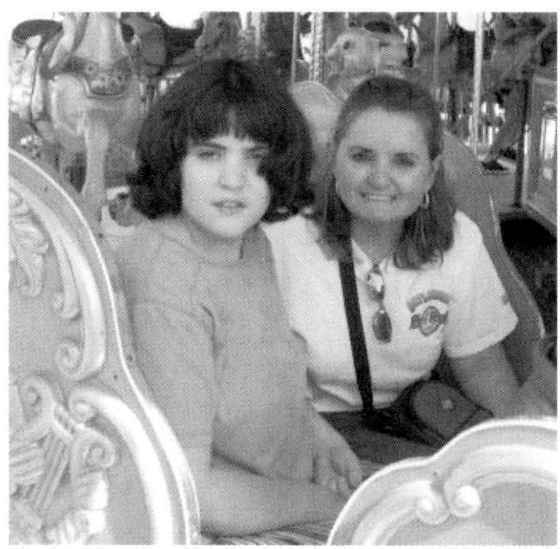

Holly was diagnosed at 2½ years

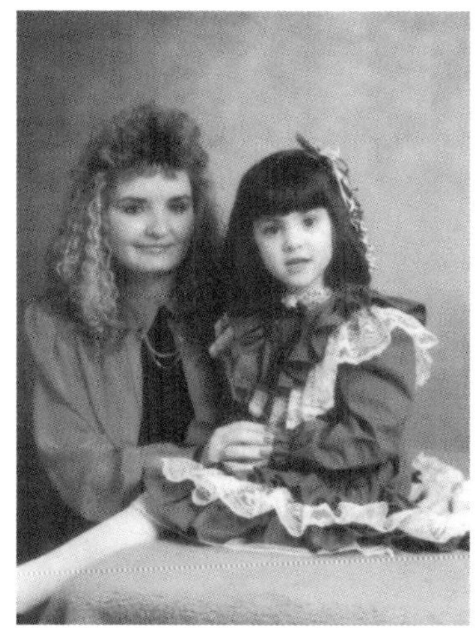

Biggest Challenge(s)

1. Placing Holly in a Group Home was the hardest thing I ever did. It broke my heart.
2. The medicine they put her on to control her behaviors scared me. Not knowing how it makes her feel since she can not talk to tell me.
3. The problems I have had in the schools that she has attended.
4. Making the right decisions for Holly, even now.

Greatest Blessings

1. To make Holly happy.
2. When she wrote her name for the first time.
3. When she was potty trained. We were told she would never be potty trained. She was potty trained at the age of 5.
4. When I pick her up from the Group Home she is so happy to see me. I feel that's her way of showing me she missed me.

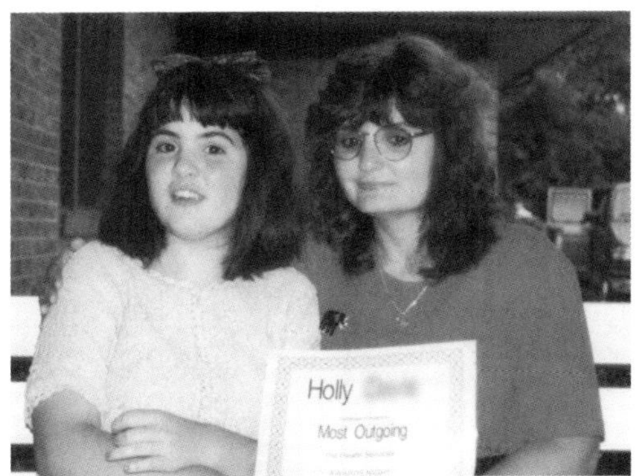

Words of Wisdom

1. One day my child will be in heaven. She has no sin in her life.
2. Knowing God chose me to take care of her.
3. She will always be there for me. I will never be alone.
4. Always stand up for what you want for your child. You are all they have.

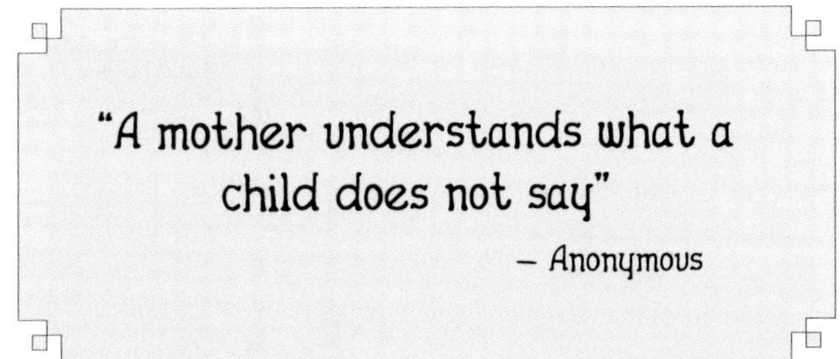

Deborah & Stacey

Georgia

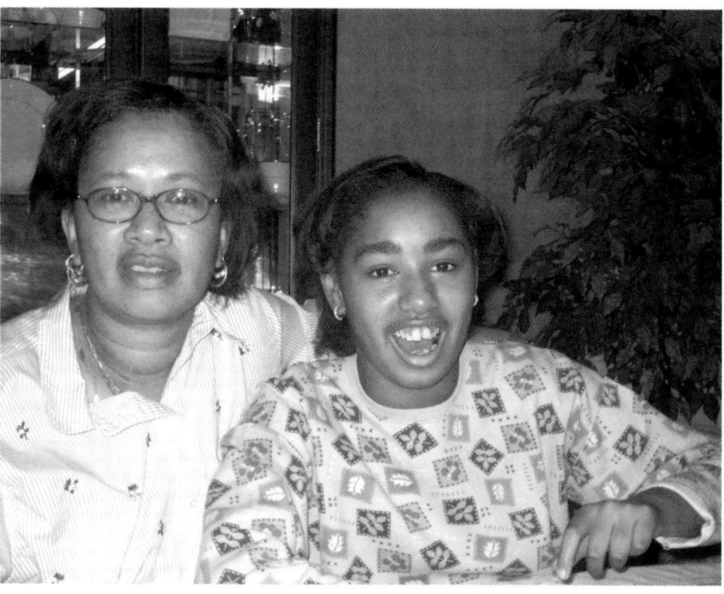

Contact:
dmajette@bellsouth.net
678-624-1692

Stacey was diagnosed at 4 years old

Biggest Challenge(s)

Our family's biggest challenge with Stacey has been multi-fold.

- Parenting Stacey through medication changes, dealing with bouts of aggression in the past, addressing severe and inappropriate behaviors in addition to advocating for certain educational services and personal support services for Stacey are all on-going dilemmas. Stacey is non-verbal which makes communicating with her almost impossible. She has minimal self-help skills, so she needs a lot of hands-on daily support. She requires basically one-on-one care in school and out in the community.

- Building trust in school staff members & respite providers has proven to be a challenging task also; I am very particular about her well-being and daily needs to a point of this being a big stresser as her parent.

- Finding appropriate summer camp and after school services have also been very challenging due to her level of care – there are not many camps and programs that will take the severe autistic population without support and that comes at a high price.

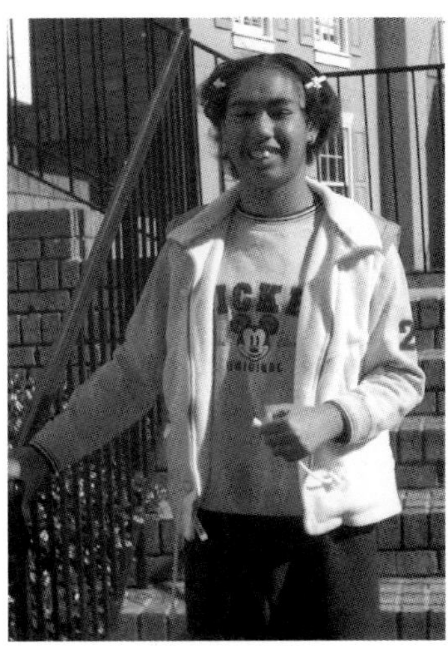
Stacey at 13

Greatest Blessings

Our blessings with Stacey have been more than what we can count. Stacey has no physical handicaps. She does not require a wheel chair or any walking devices. Stacey is now able to attend school daily with minimal issues – unlike the past. She also enjoys her great gross motor skills; she participates in an adaptive softball league (The North Metro Miracle League). She also participated in the Georgia schools Special Olympics in elementary school. She enjoys her independence when she wants to just be left alone. Toileting is not an issue at this time, and she has a very high tolerance for pain. Because of her disability, our greatest blessing is that Stacey has made us a very close and humble family. We have a lot to be thankful for. She has a loving & caring big brother, Steven and little sister, Brittany. They really adore her!

Words of Wisdom

For anyone who has the responsibility of caring for an autistic child, recognize that it can be very demanding and challenging, but it can also be very rewarding. Early intervention, education, and advocacy are key! Learn everything you can about autism – there are various levels and it's individual-based as far as the needs and the daily care. Always show the autistic child/person actions and words of love, encouragement, and support. Give lots of praise and never, ever give up hope. They'll be a better tomorrow. Keep praying!

> "Always show the autistic
> child/person actions and words of love,
> encouragement, and support.
> Give lots of praise and never, ever give up hope.
> They'll be a better tomorrow.
> Keep praying!"

Denise & Aaron

Louisiana

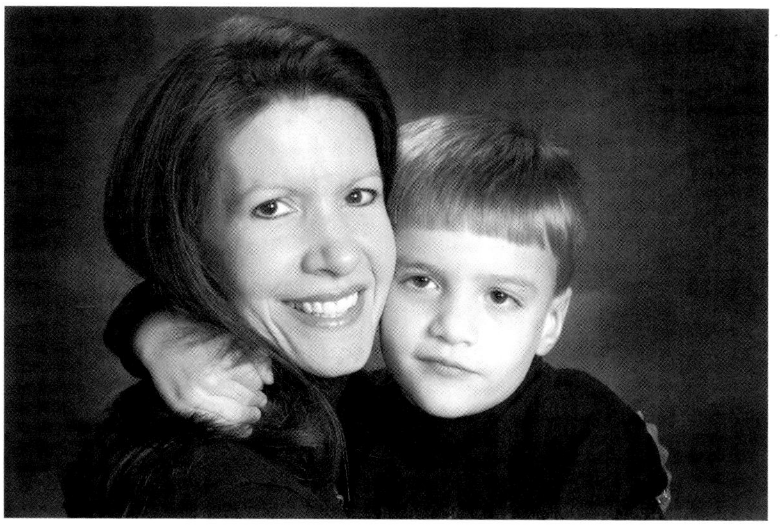

Aaron was diagnosed at 4 years old

CONTACT:
motherofboys3@msn.com

BIGGEST CHALLENGE(S)

One of our biggest challenges has been fighting for appropriate education and services. Aaron is 6 years old and was in a non-category preschool class for the last 3 years. The teachers were wonderful, but he really needed a smaller setting with more one-on-one interaction. Aaron had to be manipulated to do most everything, and if there were too many people around, he "zoned out" and retreated into his own world. He was diagnosed with autism when he was 4 and was denied services in the school that he needed. Since then he has received private speech therapy and occupational therapy almost everyday. When he turned 6, the school wanted to place Aaron in a resource class where he would have been completely lost – into himself, to the teacher and to us, possibly forever. I was even told that they were offering my son the best possible chance in life and that I was refusing it.

By the grace of God, and one incredible teacher who put herself on the line, Aaron is where he needs to be today – in a wonderful autism program with some wonderful teachers. Of course, waivers had to be signed, changes had to be made, and the school was less than pleased with the whole situation. It was a scary time for us, and for a while we were not sure what the outcome would be.

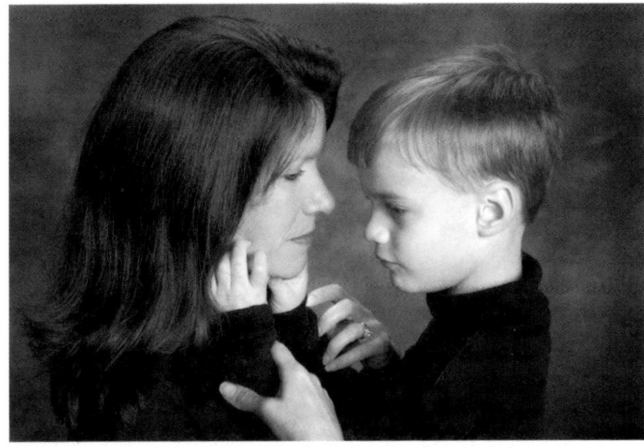

Communication is another difficult issue for us. Aaron uses mostly echolalia, or he will just recite what he has memorized from videos – verbatim. He can't quite express his needs or wants, but he is making progress with therapy. I know what he wants most of the time, but when I don't his frustration is clearly evident. He doesn't understand logic or reason. He doesn't understand that he should not run out in the street or parking lot because he might get hit by a car, or that he should not go with strangers or wander off, or that he can't watch videos when the electricity goes out, and so on. Watching him cry in frustration because he doesn't understand something is truly heartbreaking.

Greatest Blessings

Aaron himself is one of our greatest blessings. He is our second child of three boys. He is completely happy and content most of the time. He is happy just to wake up to a new day. Many times I wondered why God sent this child to me. He gave me the answer quite clearly one day as if He were actually speaking to me. I was picking up Aaron's brother's toys and suddenly realized that Aaron didn't care about these things. It doesn't matter to him how many presents he gets, how big they are, or any of the things siblings typically fight about. He is totally untouched by the selfishness of the world. He finds joy in the simple things, the way I believe God intended it to be.

Aaron gets excited when he sees the sun, the stars, the moon, the trees, or even the leaves blowing in the wind. His face is full of wonder at these things. He will stand for what seems like hours with his hands pressed to the window watching the rain, totally mesmerized. The delight on his face everyday when I pick him up from school is a mother's greatest gift. When he sees me, he runs to me, hands flapping wildly, screeching loudly, saying "there's mom", so happy he's about to burst. He throws himself into my arms with a hug beyond words.

We are truly blessed in that Aaron loves to be hugged tight, and he loves to be close and cuddle. Aaron doesn't love me because I buy him things or make his favorite food or perform some great "supermom" feat. He loves me simply because I'm Mom. His love his unconditional. I love Aaron EXACTLY the way he is. Aaron is truly a gift from God. He is a beautiful miracle of life. He is God's pure love.

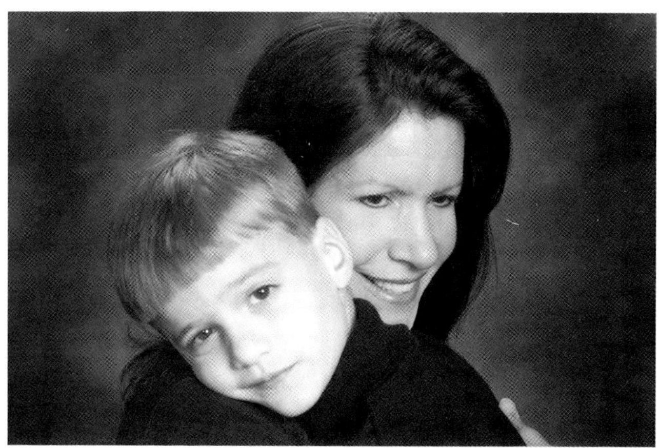

Words of Wisdom

The best advice I could give someone would be to join their local autism support group. I know many people think we all just sit around complaining, but these are people who want to share their experiences and truly help others. The friendships, advice and knowledge of others who have already been where I am going have been so invaluable to me. Had I not learned from them what I know, my son would not be where he is today. I would have trusted the school system to know what is best for him. I would have believed that they knew what they were doing, and that whatever they offered was the best for my child. Sadly this is almost never the case. As parents we must always, always stay informed to make sure our children are getting the best education possible to meet their needs. Even though our children are entitled to this by law, it is not just automatically given to them because that's usually not the easiest, most convenient or "cheapest" way for the system. It is a constant battle – one we must win for our children.

"He is totally untouched by
the selfishness of the world.
He finds joy in the simple things,
the way I believe
God intended it to be."

Erin & Brian

Minnesota

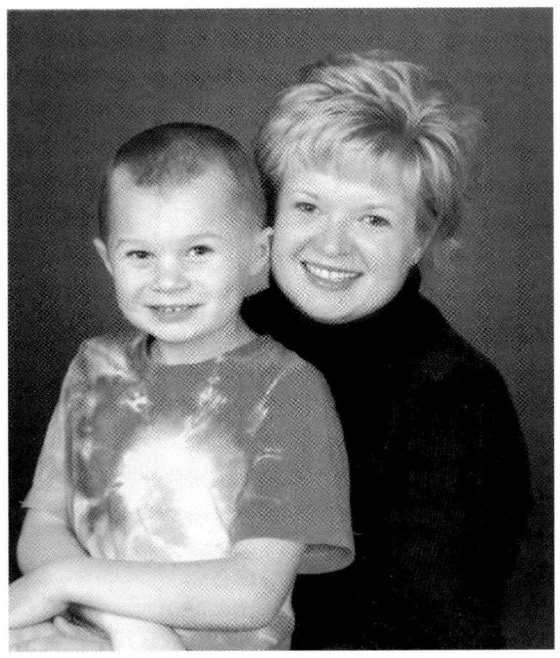

CONTACT:
erinsperling@comcast.net

Brian was diagnosed at 4 years old

BIGGEST CHALLENGE(S)

I firmly believe that it does take a village to raise a child, especially a child with autism or other disability. Finding and cultivating supports, including family and friends, physicians, therapists, teachers, social workers, psychologists, and, especially, other parents, is crucial. These supports aren't just for helping you care for your child (which is very important), but to help you. If you do not feel adequately supported and encouraged by those people who are around you or your child the most, find new groups and individuals who will listen to and respect you and your child. Remember, you know your child best, and it is up to you to work on his or her behalf!

Greatest Blessings

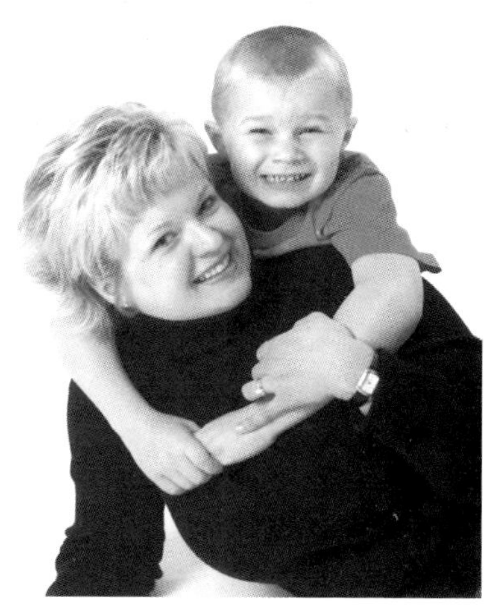

Since my son was diagnosed in March 2003, I have had the chance to meet so many extraordinary people, including parents, practitioners, advocates, and persons with disabilities, that I would not have otherwise met. Last summer, for instance, I was in a small town in northeast North Dakota for a family reunion, and there was a boy there who was very upset about getting into the community pool. As I sat with my 2 children, I quietly observed the child's mother coax the child first from the locker room to the edge of the pool, and then from the edge of the pool to the water. The entire process took about 20 minutes. Afterward, the mother felt compelled to come over to me (it must have been obvious for some reason that I did not live in this town) to apologize for her son, but that he had autism, and was the only child in the community who did. For one, there was no reason that she, or any other parent, needs to apologize for their child under these circumstances. But secondly, once I let her know that my son also had autism, we had a wonderful conversation about our children and their futures. As the only parent she knew of in her area with a child with autism, she seemed very happy to talk to someone who knew what she had been experiencing. From my end, I appreciated the support I have in place all the more as a result of this chance meeting. To go through autism as a team with parents and professionals is one thing—the strength of men and women who are advocating for their children in virtual isolation, however, is absolutely amazing to me.

Words of Wisdom

Never, ever give up. There may be days that you just want to stay in bed and cry all day, especially if your child has just been diagnosed. Even though the cause of autism remains a mystery, there is more known about this disability than ever, giving us more hope that our children will lead happy, successful lives.

Don't forget about other family members, especially spouses and siblings. Caring for a child with autism can be difficult, but still remember there are other members of your family who need you, too. Do not be afraid to ask family and friends to provide respite care once in awhile so you are able to focus on other people in your life, including yourself. Your child may also appreciate the temporary change of scenery.

The world can be a cruel place, especially to people who have differences. It doesn't seem to matter whether these differences are subtle, such as having red hair and freckles or eyeglasses, or more profound. This reality is unacceptable! Work to change that—do presentations at your child's school, confront bullying or other similar activity when you see it, or get involved in your local community or county or state government to affect change.

When parents, or other individuals, ask questions about my son I consider it as an invitation to educate them about autism—its prevalence, its uniqueness, and, most importantly, I seek to shatter the "Rain Man" stereotypes that are still so prevalent in our society. I engage in these conversations with an open mind and heart—no one is going to listen if your response is defensive. I've had wonderful conversations with people as a result—often times, the individuals who ask questions aren't doing so out of hostility, but are frequently seeking information for others or for themselves.

Favorite Resources:

My favorite book related to autism is *Elijah's Cup* by Valerie Paradiz. This book follows Valerie's journey with her son, who was diagnosed with high functioning autism. I think her book provides a raw, honest portrayal of a family going through the process of doubt, worry, diagnosis, and healing. The text is also interspersed with facts about autism.

I tend to rely more on organizations and web sites for information:

Autism Society of America (www.autism-society.org) has lots of resources, including articles and local chapter information. I would highly encourage you to get involved with a local autism chapter as soon as possible. They give presentations on a variety of issues related to autism, and can also serve as a great local source of information and services for you.

Partners in Policymaking (www.partnersinpolicymaking.com) is a state-sponsored program which teaches parents of children with disabilities, as well as individuals with disabilities, how to serve as advocates within the political system. I am currently in one of these classes, and my experience has been amazing. They also have a number of resources on their website directly related to disability issues.

I would also contact your local school district as soon as possible, in order to get plugged in to their resources, such as early childhood education if your child is under 5 years old, or with their special education services if your child is school-age. They can also help direct you to county and state resources as well, including social workers and funding opportunities.

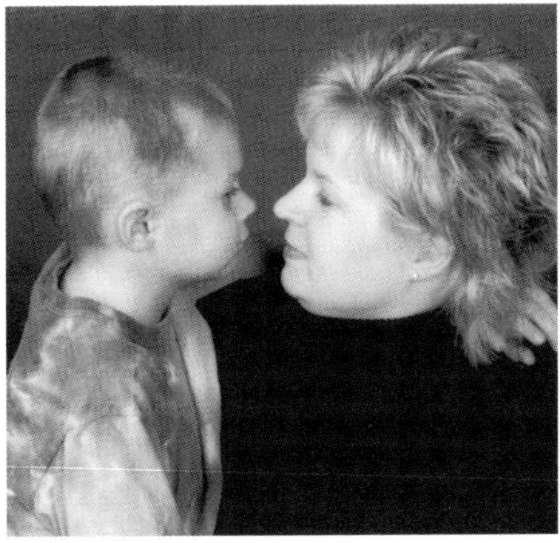

Erin & Brian

Heather & Grant

Texas

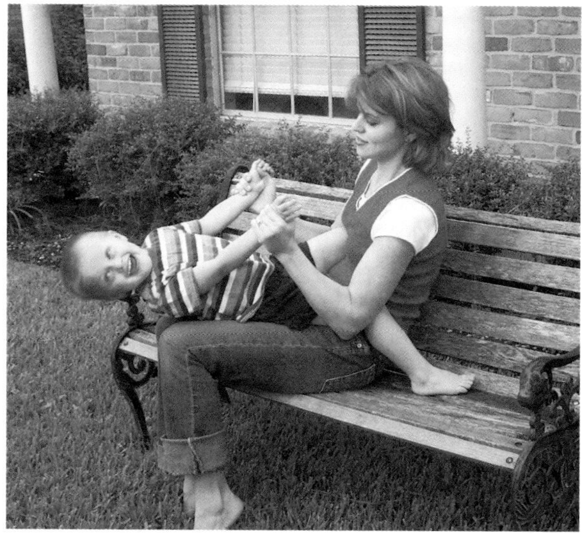

CONTACT:
Hdmgrice@msn.com

Grant was diagnosed at 2 years old

BIGGEST CHALLENGE(S)

My son Grant was diagnosed with autism in December of 2003, shortly after his second birthday. My husband and I had been informed that autism was a possibility however, it is when I saw the word "autistic" in writing that I got this jabbing feeling in my stomach like all of my dreams and expectations for my child has been thrown out of the door (that is not a good way to think).

My biggest challenge, other than insurance, was acceptance. I had the hardest time accepting that my beautiful baby boy had this disorder. After all, Grant spent the first 1½ years of his life speaking, playing and interacting with everyone. I have Grant on video responding to all of my little requests such as, wave bye-bye to the camera. It was just so hard to swallow that my son was autistic. Finally, after several months it came to me. Yes, my son is autistic. I now had the challenge of researching. I was talking to other mom's with autistic children and reading book after book.

Greatest Blessings

Grant, as well as my four-year-old daughter Madison, are my biggest blessings. Grant has a laugh and smile that are infectious. Anyone that has met him, has been drawn to him. I have had friends and family members that want to learn more about autism and when asked "why?", they say because of Grant. My aunt went to a conference on teaching children with disabilities in order for her to begin a program in her church for children with disabilities. She has only one child in her church with a disability but, because of Grant she wanted to know how she could help this one child. Now that, I would have to say, is a blessing.

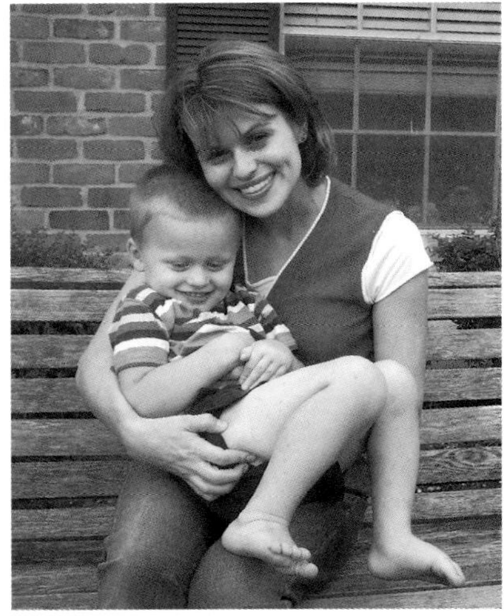

Words of Wisdom

My words of wisdom come from another mom who has a child with autism. I was talking to her one night on the phone and I must have had one of those days. I was crying and saying that I felt that I just could not do it. I said that I just did not have what it took to go through all of this. Now, my friend had always been very mild mannered however, in this moment of my pure desperation and despair she says in a very stern voice "Yes you can". I believe that applies to us all. <u>You Can Do It!</u> Never give up and never ask "Why me?" or "Why my child?" Never lose your faith. Educate when you can and be an advocate for your child. When I have told people that Grant was autistic I have had a few say "poor thing" or make some comment of that sort and I think to myself, why "poor thing", he is one of the happiest children that I have seen. Always know that you are not alone.

> "You Can Do It!
> Never give up and never ask
> 'Why me?' or 'Why my child.'
> Never lose your faith."

Heta & Tuula

Finland

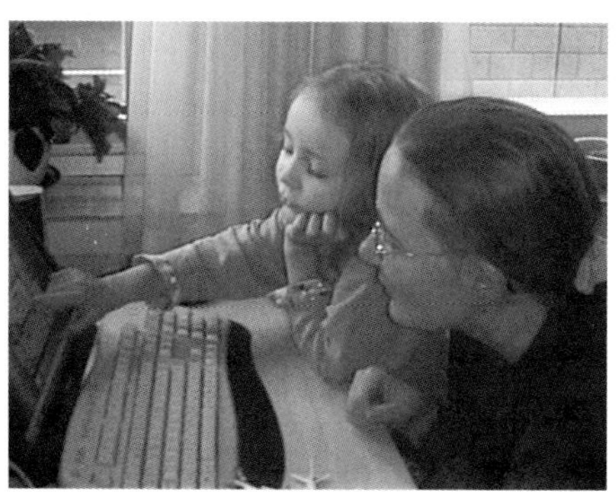

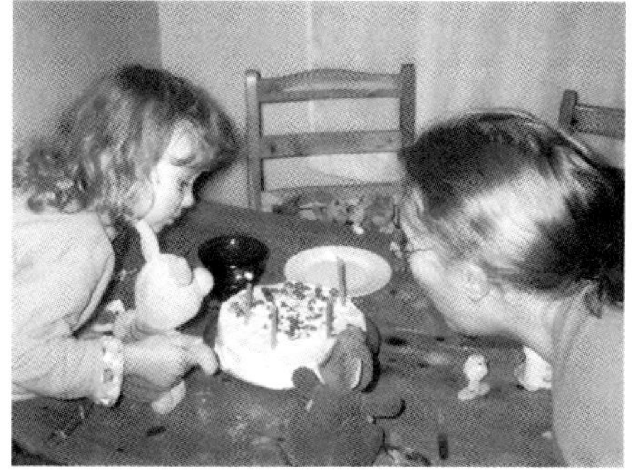

CONTACT:
hpa@luukku.com

Tuula was diagnosed at 2 years, 2 months

BIGGEST CHALLENGE(S)

I find it particularly hard to face ignorance and vagueness in people who have power to affect our lives. There's one event that kind of became a symbol for this in my mind. A few people – a doctor, a special ed teacher, a social worker – assumed that my daughter's characteristics resulted from lack of support at home. It's one thing to think that other people might be looking at you with disapproval in a supermarket; it's another thing completely to see that a doctor has written down "lack of adequate support", and put a diagnosis number after it, without ever observing us at home for one second, based on the word of other people who had not observed us at home either. And then having people pick it up, and read a list of typical AS related problems at me in a meeting, obviously with very little idea what they were talking about, telling me how worried they were. The one solution they could come up with: place my child in a children's home. This was thrown at me just before Christmas, as I was trying to make preparations for the holiday and manage a busy stage in my special education studies. I felt like I was on trial, without the clarity and structure an actual court case might have; I never knew what I was accused of really, or who had the power to make decisions. Tuula's problems certainly seemed to be my fault somehow, although those exact words are never used – I guess it wouldn't be politically correct. I asked them, "Am I also the cause of her strengths and unusual skills then?" They did not answer. As vaguely as the attempt started, it eventually ended and they just went away… The experience has left me slightly paranoid. I have to keep telling myself I can't live to please some imagined observer, I have to keep trusting my own judgement.

In daily life, the biggest challenge is her doing things so very, very slowly sometimes, and throwing tantrums if pushed to go any faster. It's OK to wait every now and then, let her do things in whatever complicated way she is finding necessary at the moment. But when you really need to be somewhere, when you are losing your one moment in the week that you could have had just for yourself – and then it goes on for another couple of weeks… there just is a limit to anyone's patience. I've had to walk out sometimes and just leave her with someone else, even when it hasn't been exactly convenient, and I'm regarded as a rather calm and patient person generally.

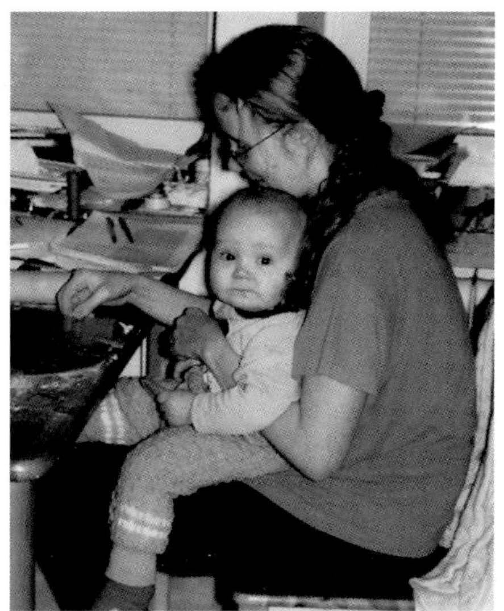

Greatest Blessings

The immense imagination my daughter has is a constant blessing. I don't believe in autistic spectrum children having "deficits" in imagination at all, just a different kind of mental landscape, producing a different form of play. Tuula is a kind of natural conceptual artist. She draws beautifully, teaching herself more constantly, absorbing influences from cartoons and the world around her. She loves to tie things in knots, and finds the most unlikely things to do this with. The results are sometimes hilarious. She loves to mix things like foodstuffs, and likes to cook with me, sometimes doing her own little experiments – does pudding go nicely with spaghetti? She just has to try.

She loves bits of string, sticky tape, packaging materials, little twigs, everything that can be used to build interesting contraptions. On her bedroom floor is a thing made out of a mangled styrofoam box, a few pens, a rubber band, a knitting needle and a small toy umbrella; a piece of cardboard closes one end of the box, and is attached to it with a safety pin and a piece of string... She tells me it's a doghouse, and indeed there is a dog inside. It's a blessing we have similar tastes for visual effects and absurd humour, I suppose. I don't mind the occasional mess, her games are just so entertaining to watch. Everyday life can be frustrating, especially when she has difficulty with transitions and does everything very slowly, but her inventions lighten up the mood. She also asks the most interesting questions, about numbers, anatomy, plumbing, anything that catches her attention. The bright, lively, unusual mind just makes up for the daily struggles.

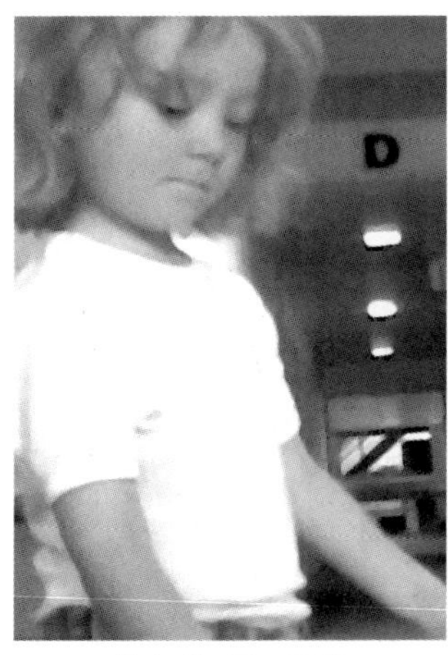

Photo: Paul Bourgeois

I'm also immensely grateful for all the people who accept us as we are: the autistic net communities I'm involved in, my local parents' group, and my family.

Words of Wisdom

Take time for yourself. Make plans and budgets to manage really getting that time. Your child reflects your moods; you are not just nurturer and authority figure, you're a role model. So think whether your child needs to learn that parenting equals martyrdom and exhaustion. Among all their needs, this is a legitimate one: to see you sometimes happy, relaxed and playful. So do what it takes to make it happen and ignore anyone who tries to judge you for it.

Favorite Resources:

1) *Women From Another Planet: Our Lives in the Universe Of Autism*, Jean Kearns Miller
2) *The Sociology of Childhood*, William A. Corsaro
3) *Autism and The Development Of Mind*, R. Peter Hobson
4) *A Real Person: Life on the Outside*, Gunilla Gerland
5) *Asperger's... What does it mean to me?*, Catherine Faherty
6) http://www.autismandcomputing.org.uk/
7) http://www.as-if.org.uk/index.htm
8) http://www.autistics.org/
9) http://web.syr.edu/~jisincla/

"Among all their needs, this is a legitimate one: to see you sometimes happy, relaxed and playful. So do what it takes to make it happen and ignore anyone who tries to judge you for it."

Janice & Amber

Louisiana

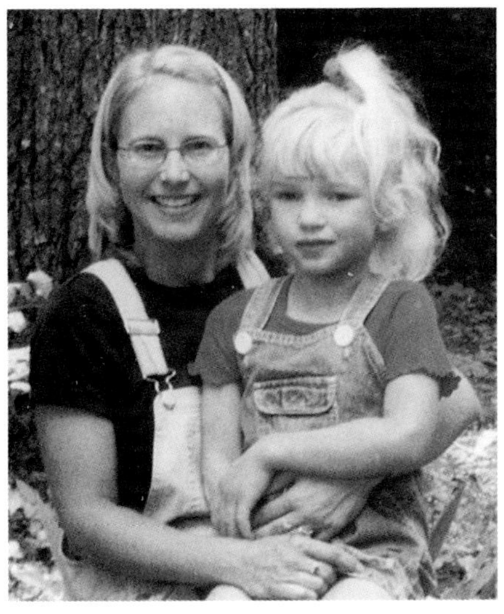

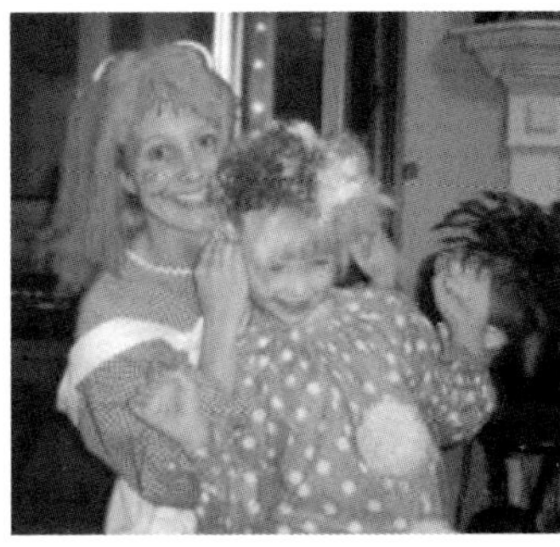

Amber was diagnosed at 3 years old

CONTACT:
mossfamily@cox-internet.com

BIGGEST CHALLENGE(S)

My biggest challenge that I have yet to overcome is being able to see other children the same age as mine (especially two girls) with their siblings playing joyfully like most siblings, at times, do. I then tell myself, "Wow, that's what it would be like IF only Amber could PLAY with her sister."

Another big challenge is finding the time and money to do the things that we think would be best for Amber. We would love to be able to hire someone to come in and help us with Amber after school a couple of days a week, OR to be able to be a stay home mom so that I would have the time to do all that a mother with a special needs child (and another sibling) needs and wants to do (including Amber's home therapy program). This also includes having the money to be able to pay for additional therapy sessions weekly. My insurance only pays for 30 visits per year for speech therapy and 30 visits for occupational therapy (which doesn't even cover once per week since there are 52 weeks in a year!), and does not pay for Hippo Therapy. (I do try and remind myself that I should be grateful that I have insurance, because some people don't or they may get even less visits.)

Greatest Blessings

My family is my greatest blessing. They live near us and have supported us ever since the day we found out that Amber was delayed. Almost always, we can get a baby sitter (our parents) to watch the children when we need. We only call when we really have something important or some place we really want to go. We've had them watch the girls for us so that we can have a nice night out together and we end up just staying at home with a good movie and each other's company and enjoy the quiet house and no worries of whether or not Amber has swallowed something she shouldn't have, whether or not she has found a way to get into her diaper and just had a bowel movement and is having a "poo-poo party" (like we call it), or if she's climbing on the desk again, etc. Our family has helped us financially also, by paying weekly for Amber's Hippo Therapy sessions, and helping us put aside money to start a trust fund for her.

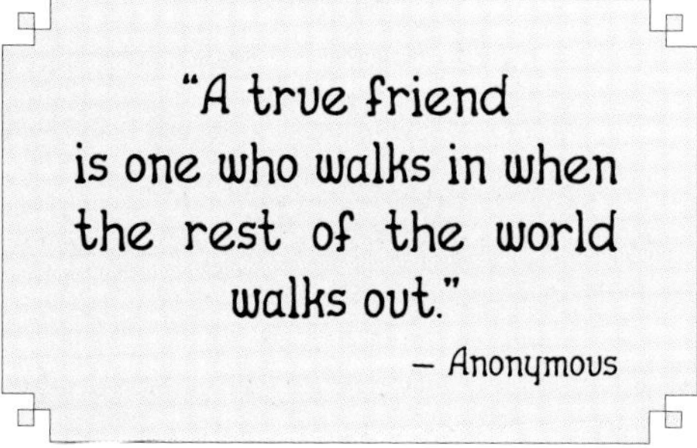

Words of Wisdom

I have a poem on the next page that I wrote for Amber. It is called "Putting the Pieces Together" — August 2004.

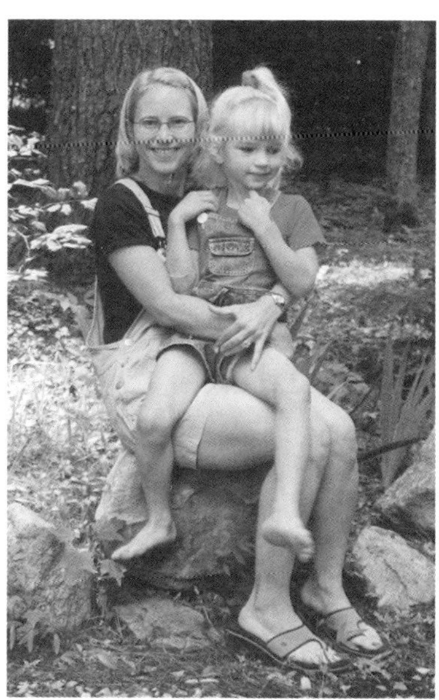

Putting the Pieces Together

by Janice Moss, August 2004

Putting the pieces together one by one,
we could never say never to our precious little one.
Our lives have changed in so many ways,
and our love has deepened along the way.

Like a thief in the night,
part of you was taken from our lives.
No more speaking do you do,
but I know you hear me calling you.

Look at me,
if you can.
My patience I offer,
along with my hand.

What a mystery this Autism is to me.
There is no map to follow, or much history.

Like a puzzle,
we're putting the pieces together day by day.
Wondering if there's a cure or treatment,
each day we pray.

We're here to guide and guard you,
every step of the way.
Whether you seek it,
or just walk away.

Others look at you with staring eyes,
but only because they don't realize,
how special you are inside.

You may not play ball, joke, or dance,
but with more progress,
maybe you'll get the chance.

Only time will tell us how you'll grow,
what you'll do or what you'll know.
We'll be here putting the pieces together one-by-one,
because, Amber, you are forever our precious little one.

Irene & Kyle

New York

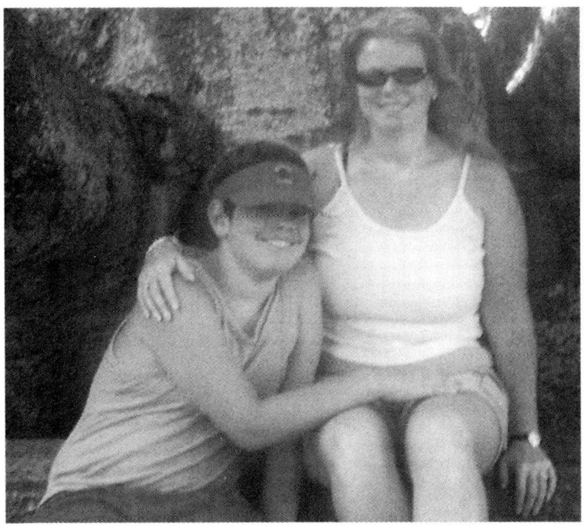

Kyle was diagnosed at 6 years old

Biggest Challenge(s)

For me the biggest challenge was to come to terms with the fact that Kyle was born with PDD (Pervasive Development Disorder), just another form of autism. When he was born I dreamt of him being an A student, being on the football team, getting married and having kids of his own. All of those dreams had to change to dreams such as the day he will speak or when he would start to realize the space around him. Now that he is 13 years old, new challenges arise, like learning to play with other children. It is very upsetting when he is with children his own age and he sticks out. Being 5 feet 7 inches tall and 190 lbs, it's hard not to see that he is different. For now, everyday is a new challenge in its own way.

"To the world you are just one person, but to one person you could mean the world."

– Anonymous

Greatest Blessings

It has been a long journey from the time he was born to today. My biggest blessing is Kyle. He is the most sensitive, loving, kind-hearted, caring soul anyone would ever meet. I would never change a thing about my son. I am very blessed to have him. My hope for the future is that he will be able to live a semi-normal life. I pray that he will fall in love and that that person will love him and not take advantage of his loving heart. But for today we just live one day at a time, who knows what that future holds but God.

Words of Wisdom

My only advice is to go with your gut. I knew that something wasn't right with him when he was born and let the doctors tell me that I was a "new worried mother." It wasn't until he was three when a pre-school teacher validated my worries. I was once told that special children have special parents. When I first heard it I really didn't get it. Today I believe that to be true. I believe that these children were born to each of us because who else would fight for our children and be their voices and educate the rest of the world except for their special parents.

"My only advice is to go with your gut.
I knew that something
wasn't right with him
when he was born
and let the doctors tell me that
I was a 'new worried mother'."

Jannette & Charles

New York

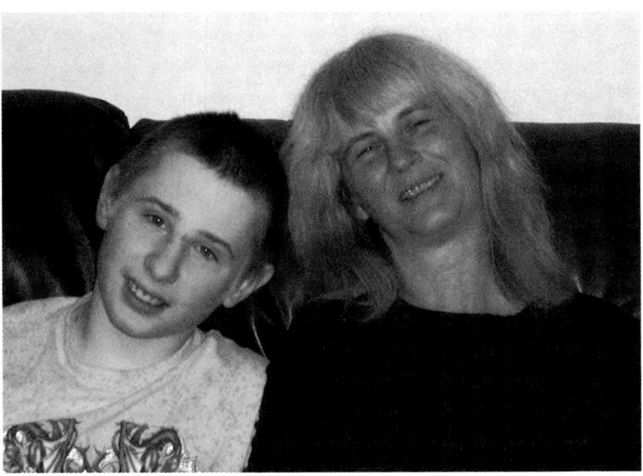

CONTACT:
js1958@twcny.rr.com

Charles was diagnosed at 6 years

BIGGEST CHALLENGE(S)

I find the biggest challenge is having people understand my son's disability. If we go shopping and he has a sensory outburst, I have strangers say to me, " If that were my child....". I use to yell at them "My son has autism. I would like to know what you tried that helped your child with autism." Of course, they do not respond. They walk away because they do not have an autistic child.

Some professionals seem to always want to experiment with something different than his learning style to see how far they can push (change) my child. This, in turn, causes overload and self-abuse problems. To this day I still fight for my son's learning style, and always will.

GREATEST BLESSINGS

My greatest blessing, other than my children, are the warm hearts of professionals from other states. They have helped me through very rough times...times that no words can express. I found angels while learning my child's changes and challenges. To Pat, of Speaking of Speech, and Lisa, at Ideal Lives, I cannot thank you enough for your support and help. With their help I turned from a crying mom to a fighting and learning mom.

To the other web sites who reached out with a helping hand, God Bless You and Thank You. Do2learn helped with free picture cards and taught me about the communication boards that helped me with my child's communications. Silverlinning, makers of *Functional and Behavioral Skills* CD, for helping with real life photos that have helped with his aggression and self care. Also, thanks to the Doug Flutie website for links that have helped me learn more about autism.

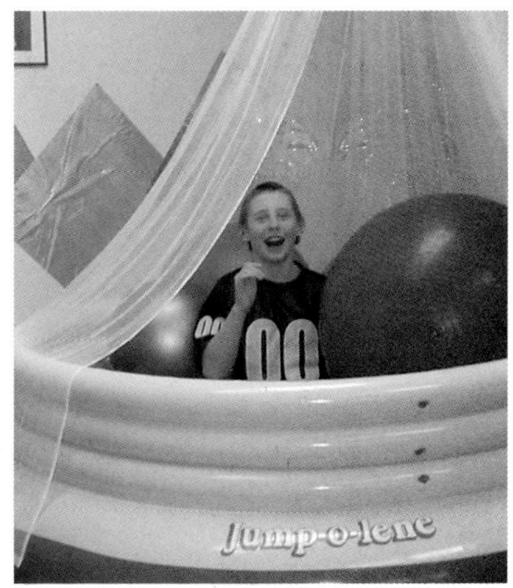

Charles age 11

Words of Wisdom

Take your time handling questions by strangers. Learn about your childs learning style and communications. It is not easy to hear words from people you do not know or understand what you are going through. Remember, you learn every day about your child, as with your family. Keep your strength in what you know, not what other people say. Know that you are doing your best and nobody can condemn you for that. Know that you are not alone. Take a breath and start a new, this day is a new one for you. The one song I think of when someone's words bother me is, "Testify to Love" by Ms. Judd.

Favorite Resources:

1) WebEd: I learned all about Autism and the differences and treatments.
2) Do 2 learn: I learned how to make a communication board and use them.
3) Ideal Lives: I learned about advocacy and got support.
4) Speaking of Speech: I got help with speech problems with their printables.
5) Doug Flutie Jr. site: I got information about autism sites.
6) OOps Wrong Planet: From Canada, I bought the puzzle he has and my son loves it, they also have an awesome links page.

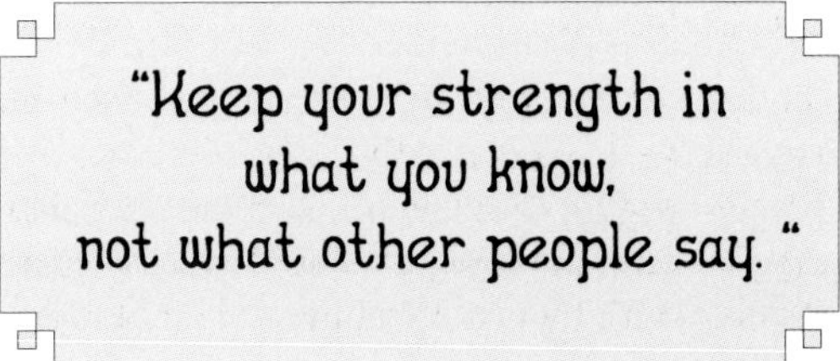

Jennifer & Amelia

Maryland

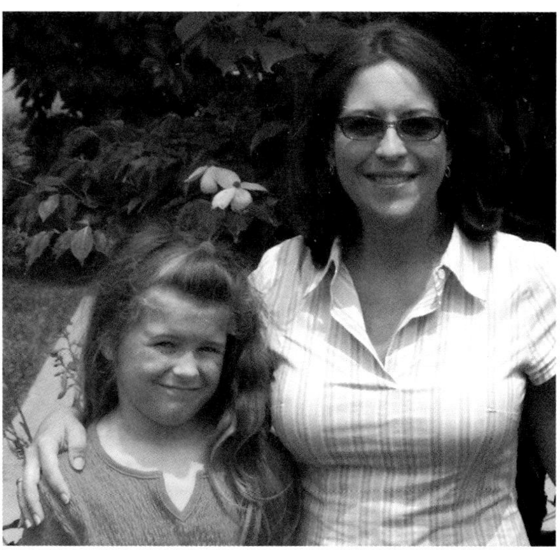

CONTACT:
Jennifer@autisticangels.com

Amelia was diagnosed PDD-NOS at 3
then HFA at age 7

Amelia, My Angel

(written when Amelia was 6)

Amelia is my daughter, and she is one of the most beautiful people I have ever known. The doctors say she is autistic; I say she just has one foot still in heaven. For now, she will only answer to "Robin Hood" and when she is stressed or in a new situation, she feels better when she acts like a cat. She cries when I use an electric pencil sharpener because it "hurts the pencil," and she loves to color on herself with anything she can find that will make a mark. Amelia is obsessed with dolphins and eggs. She regularly sneaks eggs out of the refrigerator so that she can carry them around in a blanket and call them her "babies." Whenever the mood strikes her, Amelia gives such lovely dance performances for our family. We all line up on the couch and watch her move like an angel, her body expressing the music as if it were literally flowing through her.

When I took Amelia to her first dance class, she was thrilled with all the mirrors, and began dancing immediately without music, looking at herself gleefully. The teacher waited for Amelia to stop her impromptu dance before beginning the class. "Stand on the masking tape that marks your spot," she explained. Amelia looked around the room, visibly wondering what the teacher might have meant by those

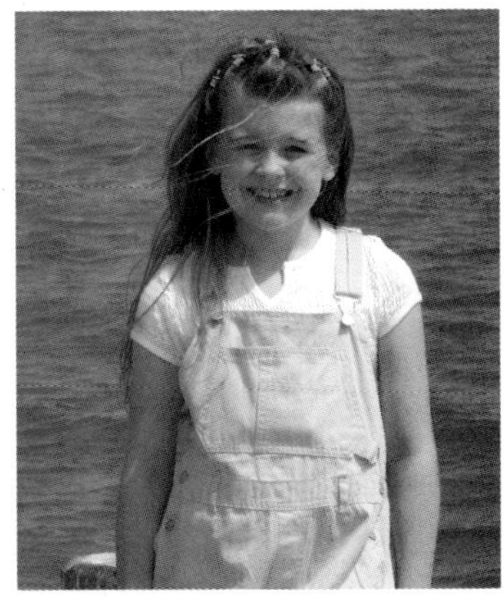

strange words that seemed to have nothing to do with dancing. Apparently sensing Amelia's confusion, the dance teacher moved so that she was standing directly in front of Amelia when she began teaching a few beginner dance steps. Amelia mimicked the teacher's every move. Even when she leaned over to turn on the music, or walked across the room to check the other students, Amelia would do these things as well. The teacher stopped several times to tell Amelia she needed to stay "in home position," which was usually followed by Amelia leaving the dance floor and gathering together her belongings. The dance steps, though no different from the moves she had performed many times in our living room, seemed to be difficult and awkward for Amelia to execute. Her face stayed tight with concentration, and she tired before the class was even half over.

I know that there is discipline in every art form and that dance class is essential for someone who wants to be a dancer. However, it is not Amelia's dancing that concerns me; it is her spirit. She may be learning the proper way to point her toe, but is she also learning that this dance is better than her own?

Amelia will always be unique. The rare and special qualities that make her exceptional, though, are quintessential gifts – not disabilities. Yes, there are challenges; for instance, she is only now learning to interpret the meanings behind facial expressions and body language. When confronted with these metaphoric hurdles, I am reminded not of the ways in which Amelia falls short, but rather of the infinite lessons she has taught me. And I pray that as she inevitably struggles to conform to expected social norms, the brilliant light that now shines so brightly within her will remain undiminished throughout her life.

It has been through Amelia's innocent wisdom that I have learned to appreciate the splendor and humor in life. I have learned that although the rocks in our driveway appear to all be gray and uniform in appearance, they are actually quite different in shape, form, and color. I have learned that there is practically no need for spontaneous language when a movie quote will fit just about any situation or circumstance. I have learned the difference between "soft clothes" and "hard clothes," and that one really can survive on only peanut butter and jelly sandwiches and Juicy Juice fruit punch. I have learned that we can make up our own rules, and that even the smallest details deserve my attention. But the greatest thing I have learned is that Amelia is perfect just the way she is. She is like a polar bear in the jungle, or an eagle learning to swim. She is an angel on earth.

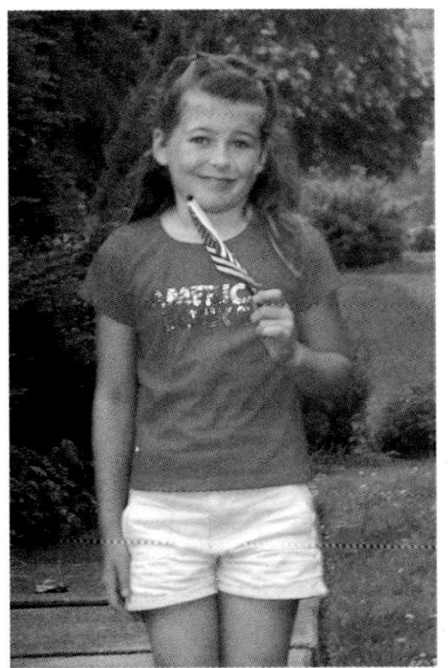

Jennifer & Ben

Washington

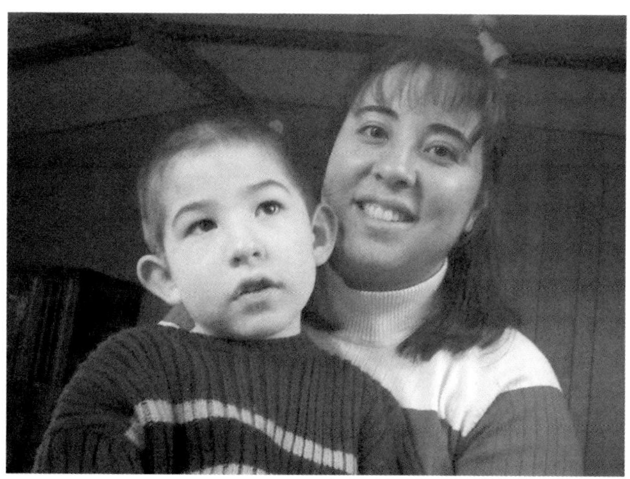

Contact:
Jennycampen@hotmail.com

Ben was diagnosed at 2 years, 9 months

Biggest Challenge(s)

For me the biggest challenge is deciphering behavior. Ben is high functioning, so he has a lot of skills including language, albeit delayed. I find myself thinking, "is this autism, or is this being 4?" Since Ben learns in his own way I have to be creative in helping him learn how his behavior affects others. Sometimes it would be nice to say, "Please don't do that, it isn't nice," and to have him fully understand.

Greatest Blessings

I believe the greatest blessings are the lessons we can learn from Ben. I believe God allowed Ben to be autistic so that those around him will learn the lessons well. His siblings learn compassion, patience, and other ways to do things. I learn patience and not to take little things for granted.

My other children are very verbal, and from an early age I heard, "I love you mommy." I waited 3 years to hear that from Ben, and I still remember the date!

> "What lies behind us and what lies before us are tiny matters compared to what lies within us."
>
> – Anonymous

> "Our greatest glory is not in never falling, but in rising every time we fall."
>
> – Chinese Proverb

Jennifer & William

New York

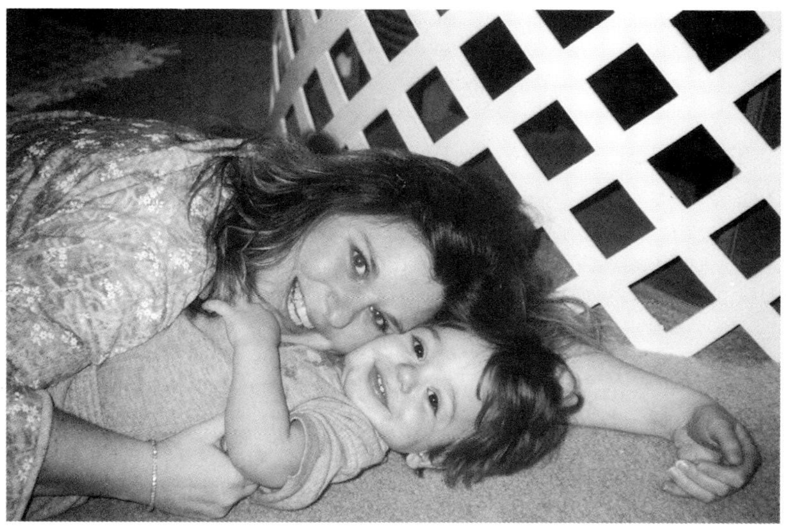

William was diagnosed at 20 months

Biggest Challenge(s)

The biggest challenge for me was acceptance. When I heard my pediatrician say that we had to have an evaluation to rule out autism, I was shocked and devastated. At the time, my son was only 15 months old and I was consulting with her about him receiving speech and occupational therapy. I was distraught that he was not talking or playing with toys and that he hated being held. I knew my son had delays, but I never expected this. I knew nothing about autism; except for a few people I had encountered who were severely impaired. While waiting for a diagnosis, I spoke to every therapist and teacher I knew and read every book I could get my hands on and despite the fact that he had all but one symptom (self-injurious behavior), I was still hoping and praying it was not true. When he was diagnosed "classically autistic" at 20 months of age, it felt like the bottom of the floor had fallen beneath me. It was soon after that I accepted the diagnosis and began working harder than ever to help my son to learn and thrive.

The biggest challenge for my son was accepting and giving affection. That was heartbreaking because I would hug him or pick him up or touch his hand and he would cry and push me away. It took me 2 months of practicing every day to teach him to walk with me and hold my hand. I used to hug him and give him a squeeze and say "I love you and you are going to love me back" while he flapped his arms and screamed. I would cry too. Eventually, with a lot of perseverance, behavior modification and occupational therapy, at the age of 2½, my son began enjoying being hugged and kissed, tickled and cuddled. He kisses and hugs all the time now and he loves it! Even though it has been a while, every kiss and hug still thrills me like the first!

Some of our current challenges are communication, socialization and imitation. My son can imitate words, but refuses to speak. He seldom says a word without prompting. He engages in many self-stimulatory behaviors, he avoids interaction with others. He wants nothing more than to retreat into his own little world and I am constantly encouraging him to use his words, act appropriately, and stay focused and engaged.

Greatest Blessings

My son is my greatest blessing. Despite the fact that he has a challenging disability and an uncertain future, he is my proudest accomplishment. I am so blessed to have been chosen to be his mother. He reminds me everyday of how lucky I am to have him and to see and learn about a world I never would have known before. He is healthy and he is beautiful. He has made me a better person, being even more thankful for everything we have. We are thankful for things that people take for granted. Every kiss, hug, look and smile is precious. Every new word gives me such joy. I look with excitement for more things, like new facial expressions, words, gestures, and learning he has new interests – like coloring or music. He really has changed my life for the better and I am definitely a better person having had him.

Words of Wisdom

Allow yourself to feel what you have every right to feel: sadness, frustration, hopelessness, and fear. Only when you deal with what you are facing can you really accept your child for who they are at that moment and gain the strength to rise above this devastating diagnosis to lovingly teach and challenge your child to become the best person that they can be. Educate yourself as much as you can. Talk to experts, especially therapists and parents. Be proud of who they are and how hard they are working to become. Always use your instincts, your mind, and your heart when making important decisions about therapy and education.

Favorite Resources:

1) The Autism Society of America www.autism_society.org
2) *You Will Dream New Dreams: Inspiring Personal Stories by Parents of Children with Disabilities* by Stanley D. Klein, PhD, and Kim Schive
3) Poem: "Welcome to Holland" by Mily Pearl Kingsley

Jenny & Katie

Kansas

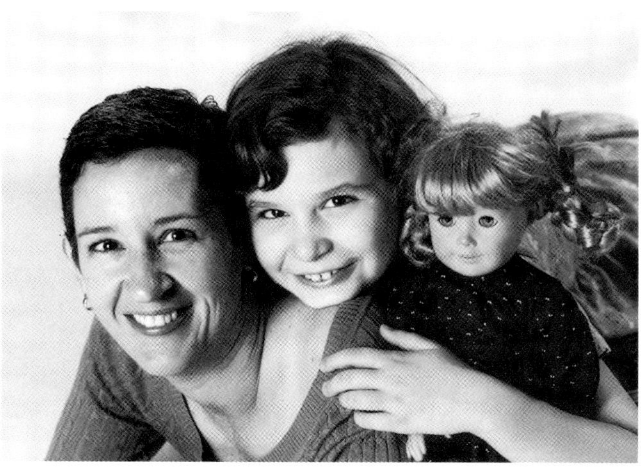

CONTACT:
wardandjenny@hotmail.com
913-385-2346

Katie was diagnosed with Asperger's at 9 years

GREATEST BLESSINGS

We are blessed with two wonderful daughters. Our oldest daughter, Katie, has Aspergers Syndrome. She is an avid reader, can't wait to be a baby-sitter and loves her little sister with all of her heart. When Katie starts to feel overwhelmed, either by too much activity or noise, she will get a book and find a quiet place to read. This always helps her regain her composure. We are also blessed with dear friends and families. Once we were attending a party at the home of some the aforementioned dear friends. There were many families at their home that evening and we were getting the grand tour of our host's new home. As he showed us the bedrooms, he leaned down and told Katie that this was their youngest son's room, and if she needed to get away from the crowd, she could come up here to read. And there stood a shelf full of books. It's the little things that people do that touch us deeply.

Katie tends to be anxious and worry about lots of things that are beyond her control. If she feels rushed or harried, she will occasionally melt down. This has actually been a blessing in disguise, as we allow ourselves plenty of time to get ready to go anywhere. It has slowed our hectic lives down, and we have found this to be a wonderful pace in which to experience life.

> "Ignore the people who are rude and unsympathetic and surround yourselves with people who love and support your family."

Words of Wisdom

The smartest thing my husband and I have done is to not worry about what other people think. Most people who cast disparaging glances our way will not be allowed to have an impact on our family's life. Ignore the people who are rude and unsympathetic and surround yourselves with people who love and support your family. We also home-school our girls, and this also allows us to set the tone and pace for our days. I am able to gear each subject to Katie's best learning style, and she doesn't feel upset or anxious about all of the changes that occur each day in a public school setting.

God has been good to our family. We are blessed with healthy children, wonderful and supportive friends and family, and a strong marriage. We tell Katie that she sees things differently than we do. Not bad different, just different. We have enjoyed those differences, for she has taught us much about life and acceptance-just as we are.

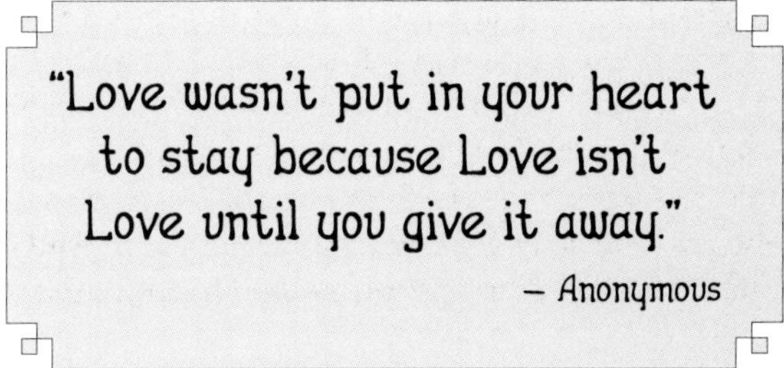

Jill & Julia

The Netherlands

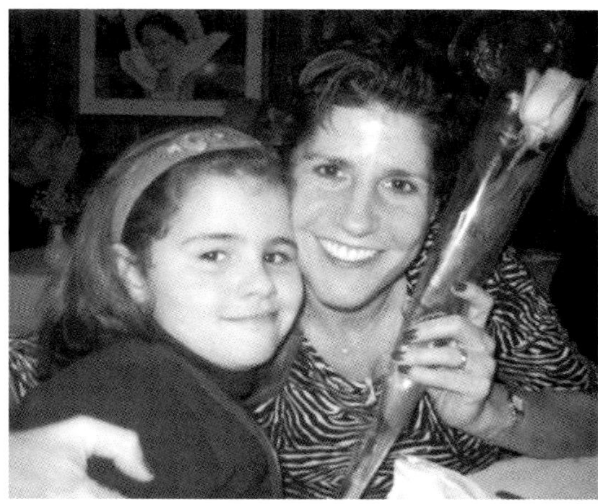

CONTACT:
jadler@ewppp.org

Julia was diagnosed at 2½ years old

BIGGEST CHALLENGE(S)

I guess the biggest challenge I have faced as a mother with a child on the autistic spectrum is separating my "drama" from hers, overcoming my pain and distinguishing it from her experience of the world. I have struggled to come to terms with the realization that I will never fully understand her, and that the best I can do is to accept her on her terms and respect who she is. Beyond that, the challenges are many. My marriage has been challenged by the intensity of the commitment that is required on both our parts to maximize Julia's potential and minimize her discord. It has been difficult for me, as an American, to be able to understand and negotiate the best care and services for our daughter in what for me remains foreign territory. Fortunately my husband, who is Dutch, has been able to be our daughter's best advocate, to get her the best care, and to navigate the intricate world of funding and services for special needs children here in The Netherlands. Further, I am constantly challenged by the struggle to accept that my daughter cannot fulfill my longing for a "normal" mother-child relationship, and that the mother-child feedback must be on another level — one which remains intuitive, spontaneous and adaptable to what she can give.

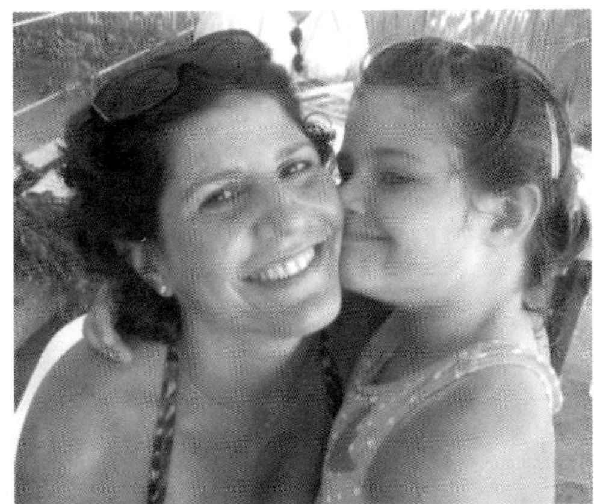

Greatest Blessings

My blessings are many. I am grateful to have such a beautiful and talented daughter who enriches my life and other lives that she touches. I am grateful to my family for their support and love for all of us, and in particular for our Julia. I am most grateful to have a kind, dedicated and loving husband who has bonded in such a special way with our daughter, and who can meet her on her own terms. He is her (our) knight in shining armor. Our friends, too, must be acknowledged. To them, she is just Julia, and we are just parents. A welcome relief and respite from the uncertainty and anxiety. I am grateful for the opportunity to meet with other parents of autistic children, to share experiences, and to exchange information. Nothing helps more than connecting with the magic of the empathy and support of similarly situated people who struggle with the same issues, hopes and fears.

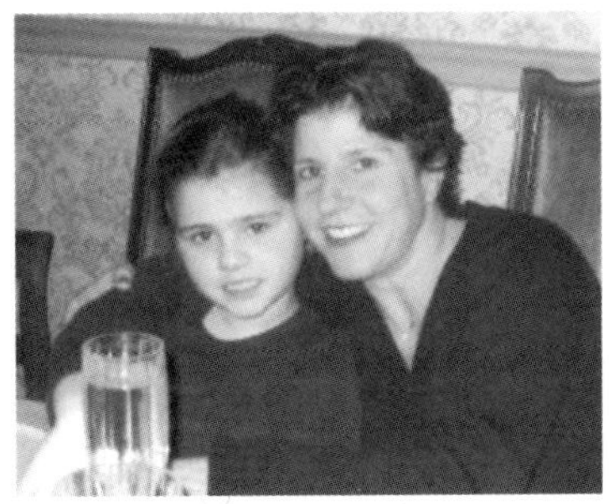

Words of Wisdom

Wisdom is born of experience. All mothers of autistic children have experienced the despair and the heartache as well as the acceptance and measured hope that our children will be able to function in the "normal" world - make friends, find a job, perhaps marry and have children, be self sufficient . My daughter is 7. I don't know what awaits us. What I do know is that I must live every day to the fullest, and not look beyond the immediate, as the horizon is as far away as we need it to be. Our children are special, and can teach us many things. We as mothers have the task of making their world safe and their path through life as smooth as possible. Like all mothers, a labor of love.

JoAnne & Joey

Florida

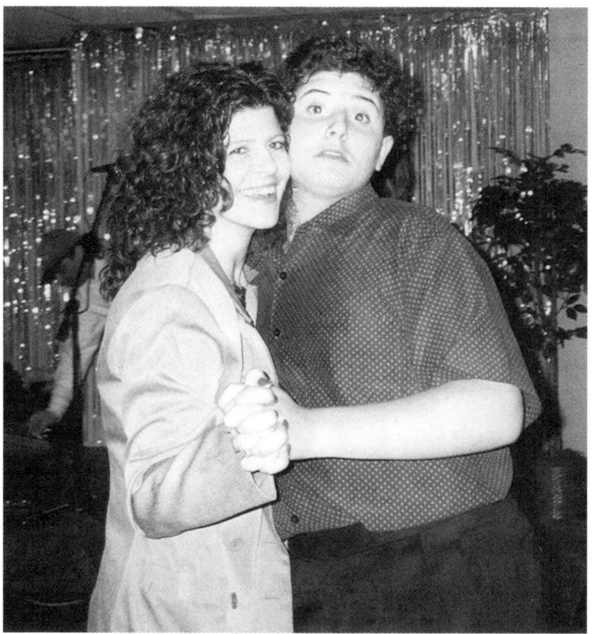

CONTACT:
autismgym@aol.com
www.autismgym.org

Joey was diagnosed at 3½ years

BIGGEST CHALLENGE(S)

My son is 19 and I will do my very best to have him live a quality life as "normal" as possible. I want him to enjoy the things everyone else enjoys. There was a day not too long ago that I realized I could not take him EVERYWHERE like I was used to. He had a meltdown in Wal-Mart for no reason and I could not move him. Everyone just stared and I had to call my husband for help, which I never had to do before. I just followed them out of the store with my head hanging down. I cried my eyes out that day. It was like a piece of my heart was gone, to not be able to take my boy with me everywhere! It was a couple of months before I would even try to take him to one store without Dad. It is still very hard, but I am back on track thinking, "He just didn't want to be in the store; just like any man!" and he couldn't tell me.

Greatest Blessings

The biggest blessing is that Joey has always been very affectionate towards us. This is probably because we hugged and kissed him constantly and still do. This was a battle we chose. He is a big huggy bear!

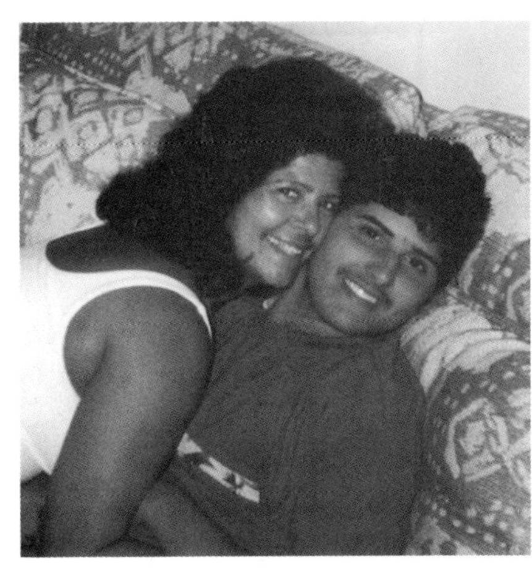

Words of Wisdom

Don't ever feel like you have been cheated! I feel like God has sent me an angel! Remember, there are more good people in the world that want to help than you think. Educate people as much as you can. I work for Disney and they have been a tremendous help to me. My son grew up with Mickey Mouse. I do presentations about autism around the property so that the employees can better understand and can help the guests.

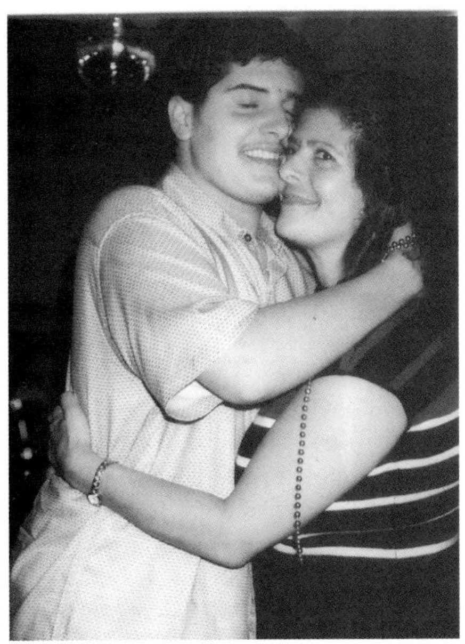

Joey & Mom, 2002

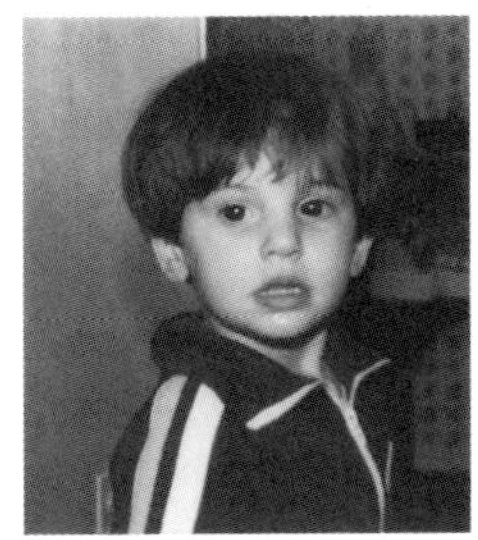

"Don't ever feel like you have been cheated! I feel like God has sent me an angel!"

Judy & Jill

Kansas

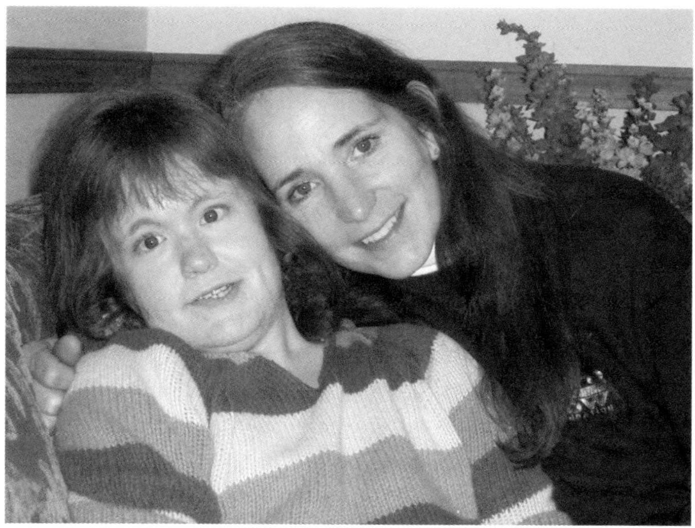

Jill on her 21st birthday, 2005

CONTACT:
Judy@AutismThoughts.com

Jill was diagnosed at 4½ years old

BIGGEST CHALLENGE(S)

My biggest challenge has been not being able to protect my daughter when I am not with her. Jill requires constant supervision and I was not prepared for the number of people whose help I would need in caring for her. Many people I trusted have mistreated her, some downright abused her. They let me down. Mostly, they let Jill down. I especially don't understand it when they are people who are in the care-giving or teaching professions or claim to care about Jill. If you are frustrated or tired or even frightened, please just walk away, take a break, ask for help — be honest that caring for Jill or teaching her is not the job for you. Please, do anything but hurt my child!

Another huge challenge is how alone I feel. Many moms shared their feelings of isolation and I feel it even more so being divorced from Jill's father. Even though many people have come in and out of our lives, the one thing I had always hoped to count on was the father of my child. He had supported her financially, but even that has not been without an emotionally draining court battle.

I struggle with my inability to influence his involvement in her life. For years I sent pictures, cards, IEPs; hanging on to hope all the while knowing that I can't make him see her; I can't make him help me out. And so my biggest challenge is trying to understand it all and be at peace with it in my heart somehow. It hurts so much that he doesn't want to see her anymore and doesn't even call to see how she is doing. Why doesn't he just <u>want</u> to? What do I tell Jill and how can she escape feeling abandoned? He has a beautiful daughter who needs him and so innocently loves him no matter what. That is what children with autism do — they love unconditionally.

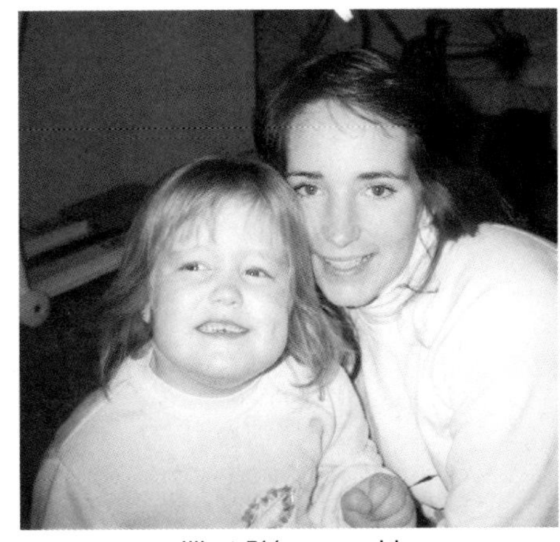

Jill at 5½ years old

As if raising her alone isn't enough of a struggle, add on the extra financial worries all the while I have to fight for appropriate school services, try to keep a job – a job that would allow me to drop everything at a moment's notice to go get Jill whenever needed, when the school called because she is sick or because they couldn't handle her, or she wouldn't get off the bus, or when the care providers had had enough; and then be there to comfort her.

Many times it feels as if no one really wants to hear about the difficulties there are in raising a child with autism. I believe everyone wants to see the me who is in control and handling every situation with confidence and determination, all the while underneath my emotions are running high. So I don't reveal very often how hard it all really has been and continues to be. I haven't shared from my heart the deep sorrow I feel from the injustices that our children face. I can't adequately describe how it breaks my heart when someone has hurt Jill, knowing she does not have the ability to communicate effectively, or appropriately defend herself. It tears at my very soul when someone makes fun of her or stares at her or makes her life more difficult just because she is different. I silently hold back the tears knowing she has not yet been able to write more than her first name, date a boy, drive a car, go to college or live on her own. I haven't shared how unbelievably scared I am thinking about Jill without me. Who will protect her? Who will love her? Who will guide her? Who will care for her when I am gone? I can't bear the thought.

I know that I have done the best I can with what I've had and I can't comprehend giving up on her, it will never be an option for me. The days I didn't think I could do it anymore are the moments I found strength, strength I never knew I had. I have given up careers and relationships; chosen where I live based on the services that would best benefit my daughter; sacrificed more than I thought I was capable of to make her life better. Still with all of the struggles, I would not trade for one moment the person I have become because of Jill and the word 'Autism.'

Greatest Blessings

I am blessed to have such a beautiful, loving daughter. Jill has taught me the true meaning of unconditional love mostly because she emanates loving others unconditionally. Her greatest pleasure in life is when she knows you are proud of her.

She does not criticize or judge you as others do her. Her life is simple, yet complex at the same time. When I asked her what she wanted for her birthday, she said "presents" which is a step-up in my mind from when she used to say 'Barney'!

I love to see the compassion she brings out in people. I don't know if she can comprehend the difference she has made in people's lives. She has given many of us a reason to love deeper, a reason to be giving, helpful and kind. A reason to pray, and most of all, a reason to forgive.

I used to cringe when I was told that "special kids were sent to special parents". For years I did not feel special. And people certainly weren't always treating me special. Then there's the 'God doesn't give you more than you can handle' phrase and there were many times I did not handle things well. But what I realize now is that we are all special. I am no more special than Marge and Jennifer and their families who have stepped in to help me care for my child. No more special than so many of her teachers and care-providers who have dedicated their lives to helping our children. No more special than the doctors and therapists and researchers who continue to find ways to make our children's lives easier.

Looking back now at all of the things I was given to 'handle' – even if mistakes were made, I learned from them. And even if it was something so difficult that it brought me to my knees — that is where I learned to pray. Even when I turned to God because I had no one else — it is then that He carried me through.

My daughter has made a huge difference in this world, for you, for me, for everyone who comes to know her. That is my greatest blessing.

Words of Wisdom

Trust your instinct. You know your child better than anyone else even though you may not have gone to school for the degree in special education. You know in your heart what is right for them even if that means you are not the one to provide it for them. I am a true believer in caregivers, teachers, paraprofessionals and even some family members being trained specifically in how to educate children with autism. That can make the difference between a good year and a bad year for your child. It was very comforting and humbling for me to spend time with several of Jill's teachers over the years and have them 'train' me in the best way to teach her. Sometimes it was hard to admit that I didn't have all the answers and had to ask for other's help, but Jill deserved no less. I know many times I babied Jill when she really needed me to teach her to be more independent. The Mother in me wanted to protect her, take care of her, and make things easy for her; when in reality I was keeping her from being the young woman she had grown to be. I am thankful for the many people who do love her and teach her every day. They are there for us because they want to, not because they have to... and because I asked for help.

When Jill was 10 years old, she entered into an intensive Applied Behavior Analysis (ABA) program that turned her life around. I am forever grateful for Kevin, the autism specialist, who went above and beyond for Jill and gave her many years of being a successful, proud student. She went from being at a school district that wanted me to hospitalize her, medicate her and ultimately, still was not able to appropriately handle her behaviors; to a school where she, with a lot of hard work and trained staff, progressed to the point of being able to sit with her peers at her 6th grade graduation and accept a Personal Success Award for her abilities, not disabilities.

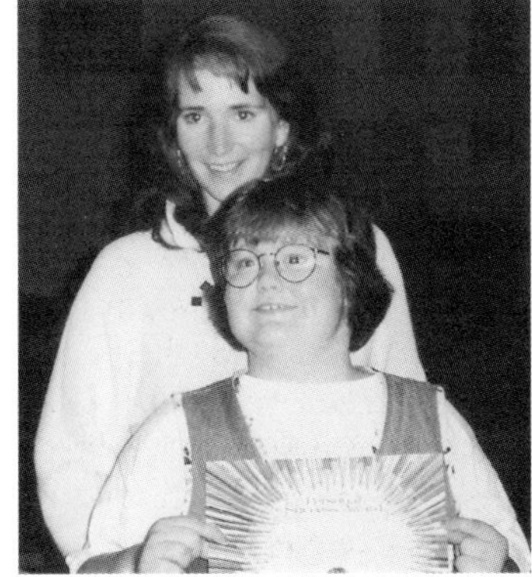

The successful program my daughter was in no longer exists as it used to, and the demise of that program is the subject of another book (because I do believe it is a story that needs to be told). Jill was fortunate enough to experience a program when it was in its prime and so I absolutely know the difference between a good program and one that provides the bare minimum 'required'.

It is important that you not allow district administrators to intimidate you. I hate to say that sometimes they will 'kick you when you're down' (which blows my mind because aren't they there to help our children?!) but let that be your motivation to rise above and stand strong. Bring an advocate to IEP meetings. Ask for a Functional Behavior Analysis and include in your child's IEP a clear Behavior Plan, outlining exactly how they are going to redirect challenging behaviors. If they are trained and educated in autism, they will undoubtedly go above and beyond to help with your child. If they don't know how to handle things they, too, must ask for help themselves.

Favorite Resources:

All of the moms listed so many wonderful resources. I wanted to list a few that were different.

There is a movie called 'Molly' starring Elizabeth Shue as a young woman with autism. She did an outstanding job of portraying not only a person with autism but also that person who is beyond the autism, a person with real thoughts and feelings.

Jill still experiences post traumatic stress from others abusing her and I feel it's necessary to mention this. There is a website called www.apergersexpress.com where they discuss abuse and adversives. Also, www.mothersfromhell2.org. Jill has had many wonderful experiences, but the negative ones are not easily forgotten.

Since the early 90's I have been involved with an organization called Global Relationship Centers (GRC). As a student, and instructor of a course called *Understanding Yourself and Others*™ (UYO), I have found not only an avenue of self-awareness but a multitude of caring, loving people who have become my friends and family. President and Founder of GRC, Bill Reidler, has been my mentor by helping me realize I can make a difference in this world by using my own 'personal power'. He taught me to see the strength I had within me all along and to use it to be helpful to others, which will make the world a better place. Take the opportunity to experience this course and it will change your life. www.GRC333.com

Julie & Gracie

Missouri

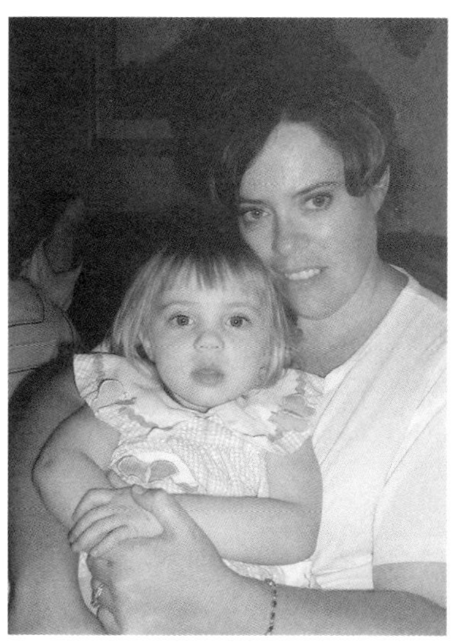

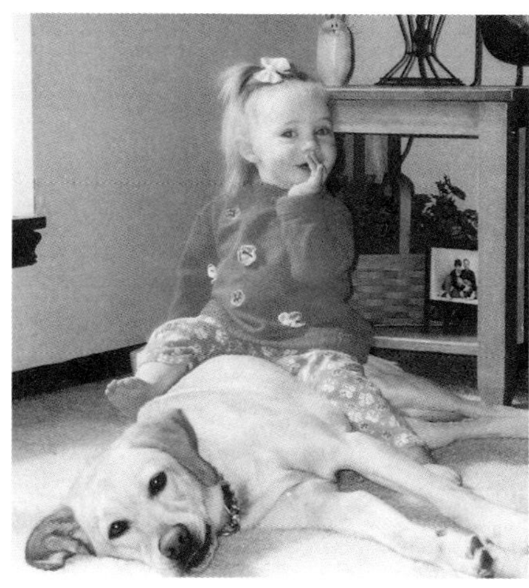

Gracie was diagnosed a 3 years

CONTACT:
covingtons@sbcglobal.net

BIGGEST CHALLENGE(S)

Having a child with autism is a challenge. I found that the most difficult aspect was telling friends and family about Gracie's autism and dealing with the issue inside myself. Having to face the reality that my beautiful little girl is not perfect by developmental standards was also challenging. Sometimes I sit and study her when she is sleeping, she is so precious, her flawless skin, long eyelashes, and kissable lips, she looks so typical, but is not. I realize that I didn't want to tell friends and family that Gracie was autistic because I then had to admit that she was different.

Greatest Blessings

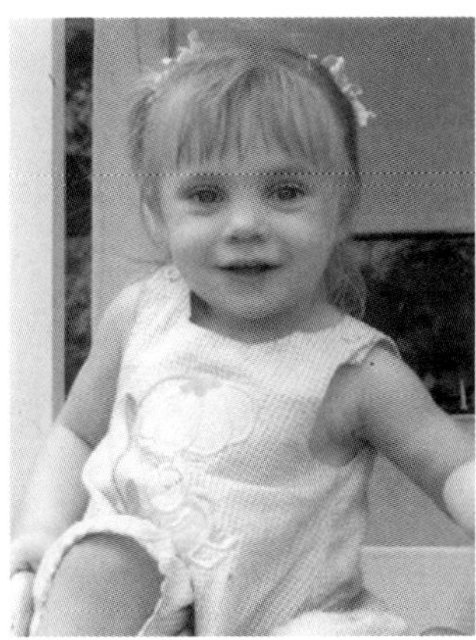

Gracie has truly strengthened us as individuals and a family. She demands that we have patience, understanding and compassion. She has brought the entire family to a place of empathy, not just for autistic children and their families, but for all individuals experiencing disabilities. We love Gracie; she is so special and has managed to sculpt our spirits in wondrous ways.

Words of Wisdom

Gracie has taken me on a journey that is full of detours and stops, I will stay steadfast because she is my daughter and I love her with all that I consist of. I still get sad because we don't play house together yet, or paint nails, but we will later. I am learning to cherish the moments of eye contact, hugs and kisses, and wonderments of a three-year old. My wise mother told me that God did not pick Gracie for us, but us for Gracie. We say that, "we have been saved by Grace and by Grace there is God."

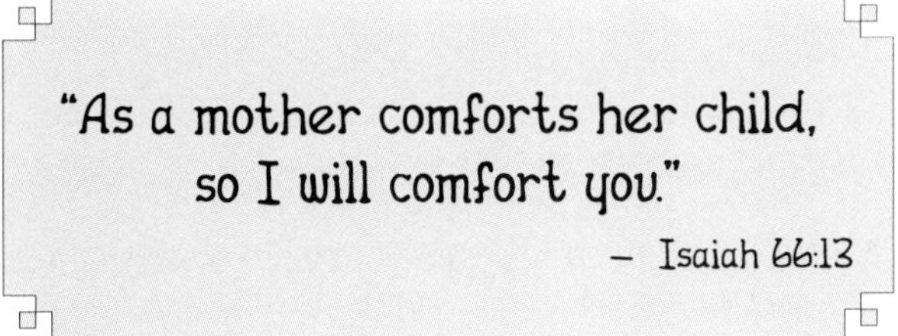

Kalipso & George

New York

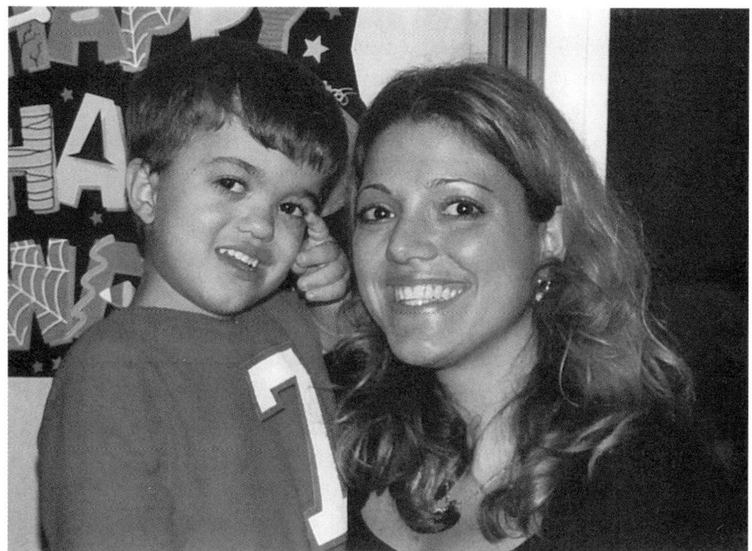

CONTACT:
kproios@aol.com

George was diagnosed at $4\frac{1}{2}$ years

On June 23, 1999, I became a first-time expectant mother. The excitement and happiness that my husband John and I felt was unbelievable. We were thrilled at becoming the parents of the first grandchild on both sides of our immediate families. On February 26, 2000, I became the mother of a beautiful baby boy who we named George after his paternal grandfather. He was absolutely beautiful, with big brown eyes resembling his mother, which I could not help but take credit for. Both sets of new grandparents, aunts and uncles were so excited about having the opportunity of spoiling him.

On February 27, 2000, I became the mother of a beautiful baby boy with achondroplasia. Dwarfism was something new for everyone in our family. No one we knew was a little person and now we had the difficult task of raising a boy who would look different from his peers. With so many questions and little answers my natural maternal instinct and love for my precious little boy went into overdrive and guided me to learn as much as I could about his condition in order to educate those around my son and promote awareness. My husband and I joined Little People of America, and got involved in our local chapter and quickly realized we were not alone.

On January 13, 2004, I became the mother of a beautiful boy on the autism spectrum. George's life course had taken yet another detour, one far more difficult than even the diagnosis of his physical condition. This time I felt like we were alone. Little people were like average-sized people just smaller and autistic individuals looked like everyone else but acted differently. Where did that leave George? He didn't look like the majority and didn't act like the majority; he was truly in the minority. I knew that from this point forward there would be countless unpredictable roadblocks that would await us. So again, with so many questions and far too few answers, my love for my darling little boy led me on a quest to abandon my self-pity and acquire as much information as possible to better educate myself in order to effectively advocate on his behalf. I joined the Autism Society of America and several other organizations providing information to the autism community. I even created Team GEORGE and walked in the Fifth Annual Long Island WALK FAR for NAAR this past fall and again realized we are not alone in our journey.

Even though in his short existence George has gained a few more labels than most boys his age, first being a boy with achondroplasia and now being a boy with achondroplasia on the autism spectrum, that is what they are, just labels. At first the labels were a little overwhelming and somewhat stigmatizing, but now I realize they are there to help others better understand who George is. To me without the labels he is still the same George he was the day I found out I was pregnant, my baby. The labels have helped identify his appearance and behaviors, but they haven't changed who he is. He is still my son and grandson to his grandparents and nephew to his aunts and uncles and big brother to his sister Maria. He is still George, the boy we all absolutely fell in love with on the day he was born. He might look different from his peers because he is much smaller, but that's okay. He might act differently than his peers and that's okay. After all, we are all different and unique in our own ways and we should embrace that instead of fearing it.

Some people say that I am strong, but my love for George has given me strength. Some people say that I have patience, but my love for George has given me patience. I truly believe that if we let love guide us in life that we can overcome our fears and life's endless road of obstacles. No one said that life was free of roadblocks, but the alternate routes that we may take could end up being our biggest reward. I have long tossed aside the road map, since I've decided the scenic route is much more appealing. Besides the highway is pretty boring and there are so many sites you'll miss along the way when you're traveling at a higher speed. I have vowed to continue to strive to make my son's ride in this road trip we call life as bump free as possible. No one can predict the endless red lights we may have to stop at or the U-turns we'll undoubtedly have to take, but one thing is for certain, when George has the green light on his side we will take advantage and keep on moving forward.

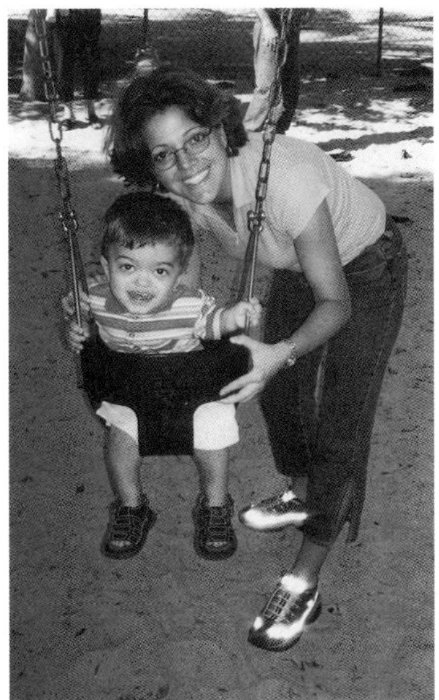

Kalma & Dylan

Hawaii

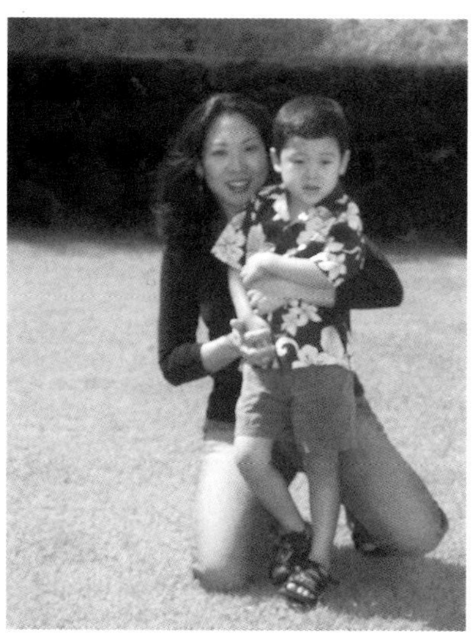

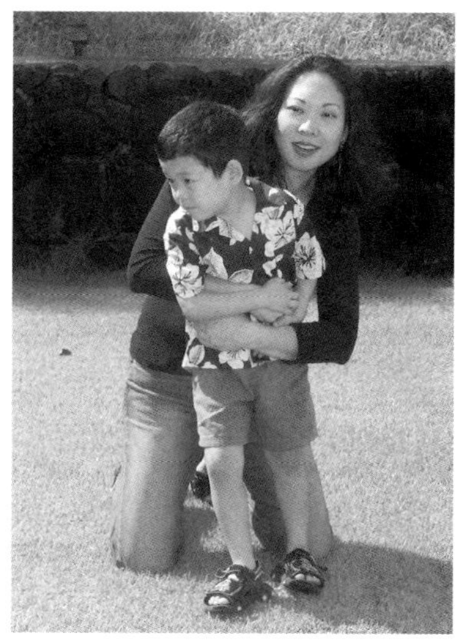

CONTACT:
kalma.wong@verizon.net

Dylan was diagnosed at 2 years, 4 months

BIGGEST CHALLENGE(S)

Understanding my child!! By far the biggest challenge has been trying to understand my son: his likes, dislikes, hopes, fears, desires. I want to know why he climbs so much, why he feels the need to chew on everything, why he puts his fingers in his ears, why he loves to smell me. When he cries is he sick, is he sad, is he hurt? I want him to tell me what his favorite color is, what his favorite food is, what his favorite song is, what he wants to be when he grows up. I just want to know him.

Greatest Blessings

Autism has brought several blessings into my life. I have come to know so many truly wonderful people because of my son's autism — from my son's skills trainers, therapists, teachers, other parents, and people who simply want to help with the local chapter of Cure Autism Now.

Autism has given me clarity. I now see past what used to be uncertainty and haziness, and I am able to see clearly what I need to do to make myself whole. Autism, which led to my getting involved with the Cure Autism Now Foundation, has given me the strength, the courage, and the push I need to make the necessary changes in my life.

Words of Wisdom

Ask questions if you have them and be sure to **listen** to the answers. The more people know about autism, the better our children's lives will be in the long run.

Favorite Resources:

1) *Behavioral Intervention for Young Children with Autism* by Catherine Maurice
2) *A Circle of Children* by Mary MacCracken
3) *Graduated Applied Behavior Analysis* by Bobby Newman, PhD, BCBA
4) *There's a Boy in Here* by Judy Barron
5) Favorite organizations:
   Cure Autism Now Foundation, Autism Society of America

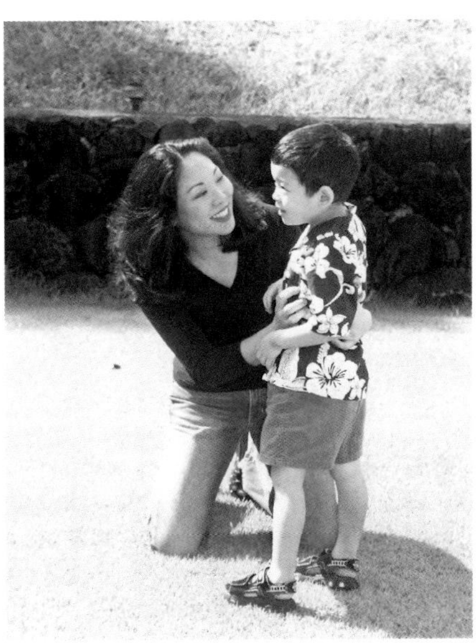

Kara & Khalen

Iowa

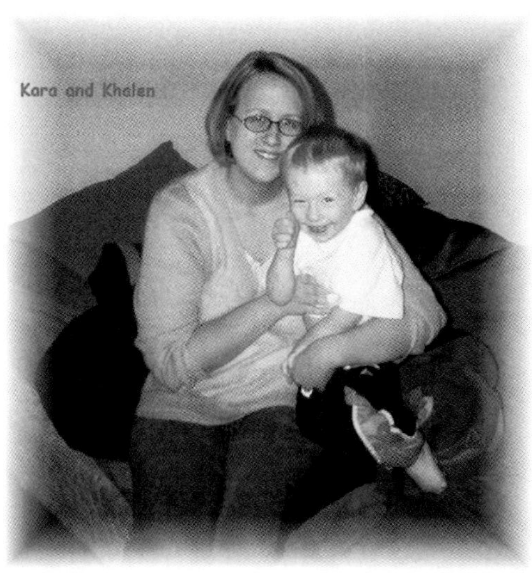

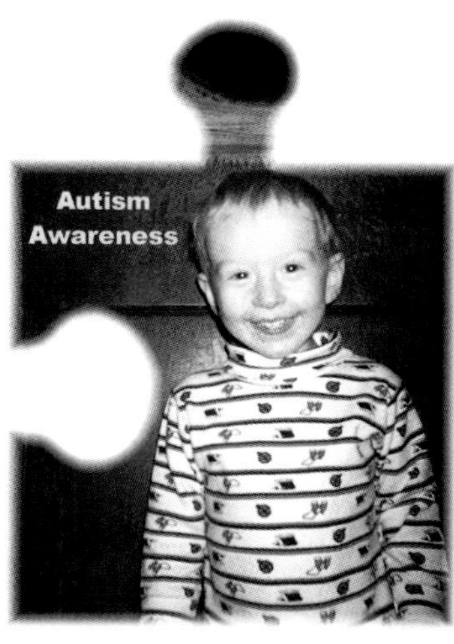

Khalen was diagnosed at 2 years

CONTACT:
karabeaucamp@hotmail.com

BIGGEST CHALLENGE(S)

For months before Khalen's diagnosis, we knew something was wrong. In fact, we knew what was wrong. It took us three months and five cancelled appointments to muster up the courage to visit a specialist. When we finally made the trip to the Sioux Valley Children's Specialty Clinic in Sioux Falls, South Dakota our hopes were still high. Yet when they returned with the diagnosis of autism we were devastated. "No, not us, not him, they can't be right. Our perfect little boy could not have a disability."

It took us several months to realize that while he was text-book disabled, he was still our perfect little boy. We had to get over our feelings in order to help him become the best person he can be.

To this day we still have confused, hurt and angry days. Some people just don't know what is like to have their child but never have a conversation with them.

Greatest Blessings

Our greatest blessing was an early diagnosis. Since then, he has excelled in a structured educational setting, whether at home, day-care or school. We are very fortunate to have excellent support through the local AEA with caring professionals who want nothing more than to see our son succeed in life. And he will.

Words of Wisdom

Cherish every word that comes out of their precious little mouths – yes even the dirty ones. I realized that even though Khalen seems to be in his own little world at times – at least it is a happy one and he does not fear the things I fear. Take time for yourself, a good mother is a happy one. Disability is only a text book word. Take negative comments as an opportunity to educate people on autism.

Favorite Resources:

1) Support Group: http://groups.msn.com/AutismSupportGroup
2) Moms on a Mission for Autism: http://www.momsonamissionforautism.org/
3) National Alliance for Autism: http://www.naar.org/
4) Autism Society of America: http://www.autism-society.org
5) Autism Society of Iowa: http://www.autismia.org/

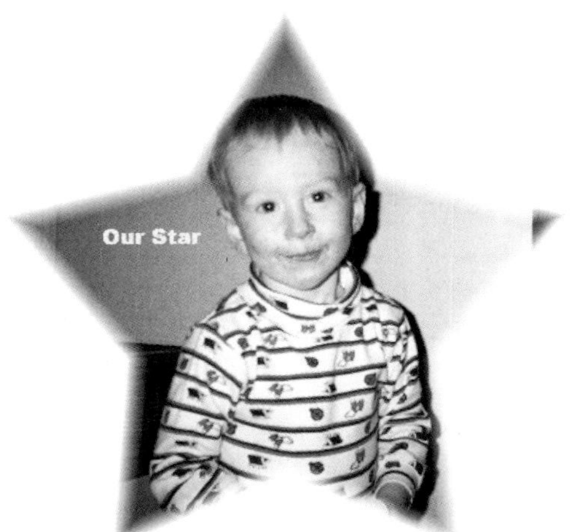

"Disability is only a text book word. Take negative comments as an opportunity to educate people on autism."

Kara & Kyle

Louisiana

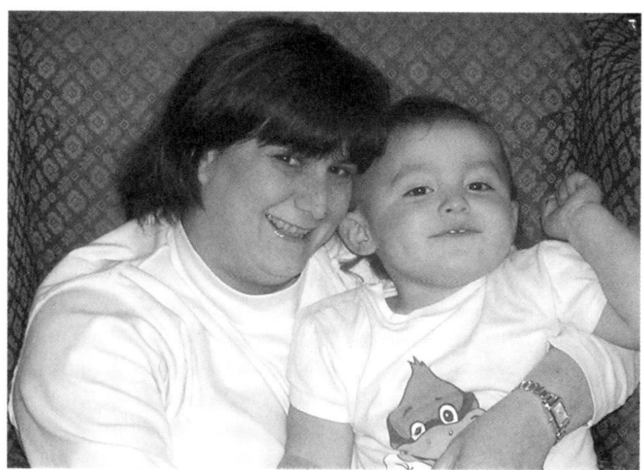

CONTACT:

Tobasco1@cox.net

Kyle was diagnosed at 30 months

What I've Learned

My gut instincts told me something was not right with Kyle's development long before the first evaluation. All of the old wives tales were thrown at us; his sister is talking for him, boys are always slower than girls. It took a year and two months to get the diagnosis of autism. Kyle had more evaluations and procedures than I care to remember. One doctor said he was not on the spectrum and another expert said he was. Some of the therapist agreed, others did not. In that time our lives changed in a way we never dreamed possible.

Fear takes on many forms depending on the person it strikes. My husband was in denial, while I took the education route. I never stopped to address my feelings, I just dove head-on into all of the information I could get my hands on at the time. I joined an online support group which proved to be my saving grace. Next, I wanted a local support group and when none could be found, I formed my own. This was my coping mechanism. In my mind, the more knowledge I had and the busier I stayed, the less pain I would feel if I could just stay one step ahead of this disorder that stole my dream child.

This past year I have felt the saddest of my life, yet I have also felt the greatest joy of my life. My dream child was just that and my heart broke. My happiest moment was when I realized the Kyle in front of me surpassed any accomplishment my dream child could have ever reached. My Kyle is the most precious little boy in the world and the happiest child I have ever encountered. He may have delays, but he is not the least bit bothered by them.

As I watch him struggle to advance in his development, I also see the joy that comes from each new discovery he makes. He has taught me to slow down and enjoy the little things. He has taught me that he will get there in his own time. This is the most precious gift I have ever received.

Throughout this past year I learned what depths a "mother's love" can reach. I have learned that I am strong enough to be the mother of a child with a disability. I have learned that I will stop at nothing to get what my son deserves and what is guaranteed by law. I have learned that some people are ignorant and wear it on their sleeve for everyone to see, while others are angels sent to support you just when you need them. I have learned that I cannot fight this alone. I have learned to give this to God and in return He has showed me the path I need to follow. I have learned that Kyle is autistic.

"I have learned that I am strong enough to be the mother of a child with a disability."

Kori & Cole

Washington

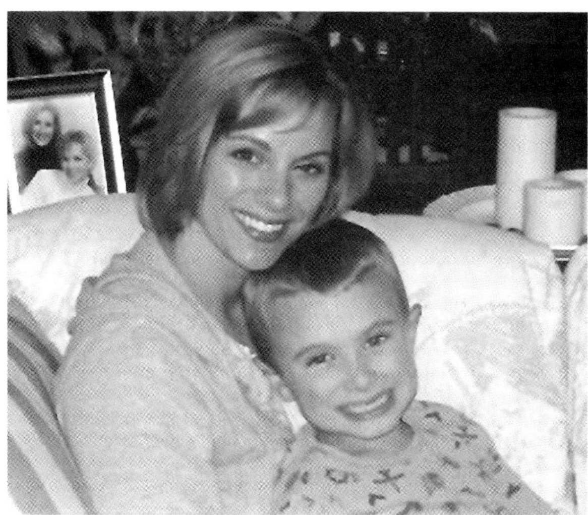

CONTACT:
kori_gaddis4@yahoo.com

Cole was diagnosed Asperger's at 6 years

BIGGEST CHALLENGE(S)

For me, one of the biggest challenges is simply trying to figure out how to parent my son. You just cannot parent an autistic child the same way you do a neuro-typical child. It involves a lot of trial and error and it changes with all the different ages and stages our children go through. There aren't many parenting books I can relate to, and I rely a lot on parents who are further down the road than I am. They are full of ideas, and words of encouragement.

Another challenge is dealing with isolation…my son's isolation and our family's isolation. As Cole gets older, the difference between Cole and other children his age becomes amplified. He does not get invited to birthday parties like other kids, and he doesn't get invited to play. He is often on the outside looking in and it is painful to watch. I've also noticed that people I've been friends with for a long time call less frequently. I know it's because they do not understand our challenges, but it still can be painful, and lonely.

I believe our biggest challenge, however, is ensuring that our son has a fulfilling childhood, and that he grows into his brightest potential. He is incredibly smart, and loving, and I want the world to know it!

Greatest Blessings

We have been blessed in so many ways. First and foremost we have a family that love and support Cole no matter what. We have a few close friends that also love Cole, and his autism is not even a consideration. If love alone could cure autism, Cole would be completely recovered!

We are also blessed with a wonderful school and staff. I know so many families that struggle with their school districts and it breaks my heart. School is such a big part of life! Cole's teachers are exceptional and dedicated and we are lucky to have them. That doesn't mean that school is easy, but it does help to have teachers that understand autism and the many challenges autistic children face.

Our greatest blessing, however, is Cole. He is loving, and sweet, and so bright. When he laughs it comes from deep in his belly, and it is truly infectious! He is a joy!

Words of Wisdom

When a family first gets the diagnosis of autism, one of the first responses is to want to read everything, and learn everything and just submerge oneself in all things pertaining to autism. And you want to try all the treatments possible all at the same time. Well, this is a life long journey, and there is lots of time to learn everything you need to learn. There is so much information and it is often overwhelming to sort through it. Take a deep breath and slow down.

Something that I found to be helpful in facing my son's diagnosis was taking time to "mourn." Like any parent, I had so many hopes for Cole's future. A diagnosis of autism often means many hopes and dreams you had for your child have been altered. You just have to shift your expectations and create *new* dreams.

Most importantly, find other parents like you, whether it's through your school district or a local support group. It helps you feel less alone, they offer support that no other group of people could possibly offer, and they are often the best resources. Eventually, as you travel down the road, your own experiences will be helpful to another family just beginning their journey, and that is extremely rewarding!

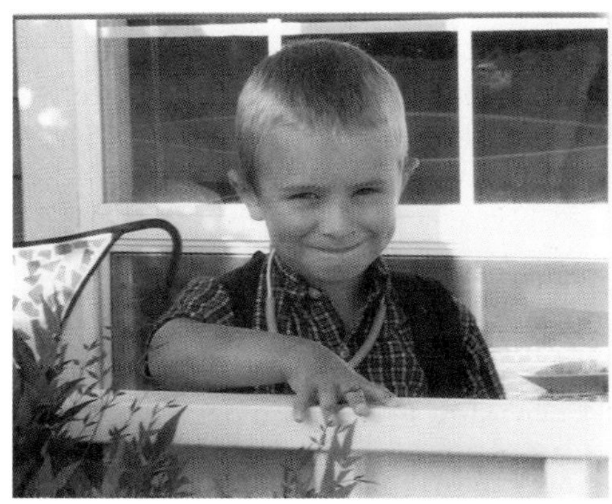

Kris & Robbie

Kansas

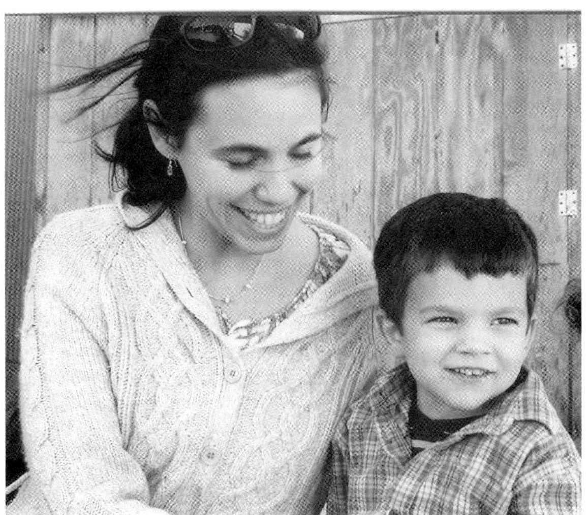

CONTACT:
kpjive@hotmail.com

Robbie was diagnosed at 3 years, 2 months

BIGGEST CHALLENGE(S)

When I found out that my son was diagnosed with autism, I suppose the biggest challenge was facing the fact that life was going to be very unpredictable and that it was going to take a lot more strength and self-discipline to be a good parent. I had always had a relatively easy and stable life. I had been fortunate to grow up in a loving family largely free of trauma or loss. I was smart enough, and found school (and later graduate school) fairly easy. I had actually worried that perhaps my first big let-down in life would be the inability to conceive children at all. So, when Robbie was conceived, I was thrilled. I had a beautiful healthy daughter 20 months later and honestly could not believe my luck. So, as strange as it may sound, when Robbie was diagnosed, my first thought was, "Well, here it is. Here is the challenge that fate was simply waiting to hand out."

I never once thought to myself, "Why me?" Just the opposite, I immediately took it as my cross to bear, feeling armed with a wonderful husband and supportive extended family. Furthermore, I had already fallen in love with Robbie and no diagnosis could change that. However, what followed (and continues to this day) is this aching, ever-present anxiety about what I am or am not doing at any given moment. It's the balancing act of trying to live a "normal life" without overlooking any possible intervention that could help him. How do I work 40 hours a week, fulfill the role of a wife, fulfill the role of mother to a typically developing very active two-year old, and still give Robbie everything that the experts say we should be giving him? There are simply not enough hours in the day, and I hold myself in contempt whenever I get too tired to be my best. That is one of the most frustrating things.

Coming in close second, is the absolute disdain at the thought of anyone pitying me or my family. It enrages me to think that anyone may think, "Poor Kris, poor Robbie, what they must go through…" The fact is that we go through a lot, but do people *really* know that I think my son is the best boy on the planet, autism and all, and that I wouldn't trade places with anyone? Do they really understand the profound love I have for him and an appreciation for all he is teaching me about life? I am the lucky one because Robbie is my kid.

Greatest Blessings

The greatest blessings in my life, next to the kids themselves, are without doubt my husband and my parents. When I watch Paul interact with Robbie and his sister, I think that I must have been the smartest woman in the world when I married him. The truth is that he is more patient, more loving, more genuine, and more involved than I am sometimes. He leaves me alone when I am weeping about things and is just there for all of us, ever present, and ever stable. Paul is a professional drummer and one interesting twist of fate is that Robbie's perseverations include drums and the Beatles. At ten months old, Robbie clung obsessively to drum sticks as if his soul was connected to Paul's from the beginning of time. Today, if one were to identify a "savant skill" of Robbie's, drumming would be it. He can do "triplets" on the snare drum, keep a beat, and loves "playing with the band." Robbie's grandparents (both my parents and his paternal grandmother) have been a huge blessing. They love and accept him, never judge what we are doing in terms of interventions, and always offer their full support. Just knowing that they are there is such a comfort.

Words of Wisdom

It would be presumptuous of me to think I have much to offer in terms of wisdom to others. The main thing is not to compare your child to other children, or your family to other families. Once you free yourself and your child of the burden of living up to any predetermined norms, it gets easier. You look at the situation and say, "Here is the hand I have been dealt. I can fuss about it, but I can't change the facts." All you can change is how you are going to respond to those realities and live well within them. This is easy for me to do when I look at Robbie, because I think he is so cool. It's harder to do when I look at myself and constantly wonder about my parenting. At the same time, it is all too easy to get into "information overload" and forget the point of all of the parenting tips, interventions, and approaches. One thing I know for sure is that I will *never* spend more time on the Internet trying to find the right answers than I spend playing with my son. I might not get it perfect, but at least he will have lots of memories of us being together.

"Once you free yourself and your child of the burden of living up to any predetermined norms, it gets easier."

Kristin & Colin

New Jersey

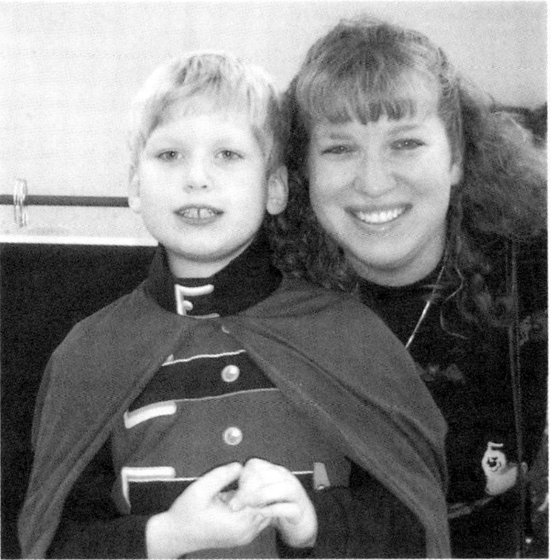

Colin age 7

Colin was diagnosed at 26 months

Biggest Challenge(s)

I think that challenges continue to arise as children grow, typical or not, but the challenges you face when your child has special needs can be much more difficult to solve or overcome. Some of these challenges are within you and some of them have to do with the outside world. It is a challenge to accept the fact that your child has been diagnosed with autism and as much research as you do about this disorder, no one has the answers. You cannot find out what causes autism and you do not know exactly what this diagnosis means for your child. I kept going over and over every detail of my pregnancy, his birth, his infancy, and our family trees, looking for answers. I researched everything – every theory on cause and every treatment available. I would have given anything for a crystal ball to tell me what his future holds. I still do all of these things, just to a much lesser degree. Instead I focus my energy on my child's individual needs and what I can do for him now, regardless of the uncertainty.

It is a challenge going out in public and not knowing how your child is going to behave or if he will like or dislike where you are going, even the fun places – like an amusement park. This challenge has also gotten easier. Colin has become much more agreeable and I have learned to prepare for these outings: bring along a game or snack, tell your child what you are going to do (social story), and when necessary, educate the general public (or just ignore their reactions).

It is a challenge to feel like you are ever doing enough. It is a challenge to read through all of your options and feel that you are making the right decisions. It is a challenge to find enough therapists and hours for treatment, particularly when the child is not yet old enough for school. It is a challenge to find appropriate childcare where you feel people understand your child and he will be safe and happy. It is a challenge to figure out what is wrong when your child is sick and to find a doctor who you trust to do this. It is a challenge to spend equal quality time with your child with autism and his sibling. It is a challenge to send your child places without you, when they cannot report to you about what has happened in their day – good or bad (particularly school and visitation to his father's). It is a challenge to do all of these things as a single, working parent. It is a challenge to find the time, money, and energy for all of these things.

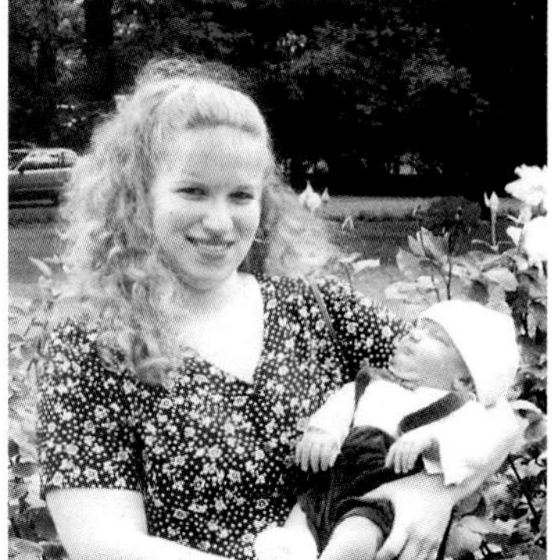

1997

Greatest Blessings

I am so blessed to have two beautiful, smart, loving children! I love my children with all of my heart and soul – they are my world. Regardless of all of the challenges, when they give me a hug, when they smile, when they do something cute, when they have fun, when they sleep like little angels – my heart melts! I celebrate every success, every step along the way, no matter how big or small. The little things that come so naturally to most children can take a long time and a lot of effort for Colin. Learning to greet people and remembering their names, being able to communicate what he wants or doesn't want, potty training, trying new foods, answering questions, using a computer mouse, playing a game, getting dressed, having a conversation, and the list goes on and on.

I am blessed to have a daughter who is loving and patient with her brother. She is twenty-two months younger than him and has grown up with a natural talent to interact and communicate with him. She is patient to wait for a response and to persevere without one. She also recognizes his accomplishments and is excited about them. It is a blessing to watch her grow and to see how she absorbs everything about her environment!

I am blessed to have family and friends who support us both emotionally and by lending a helping hand. I do not want pity; I just want to feel love and acceptance. It is such a blessing when people try to get to know Colin and realize how truly amazing he is.

Words of Wisdom

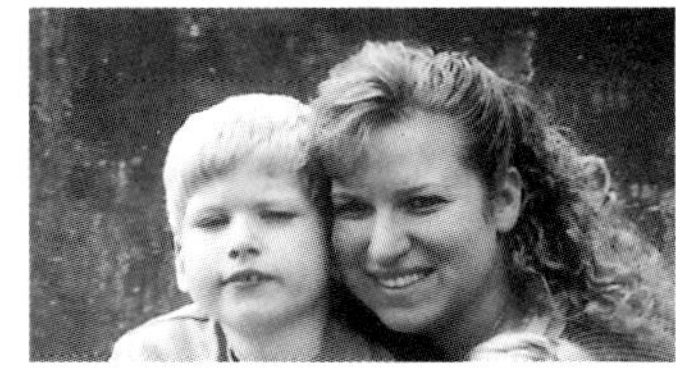

- Do not get caught up in the label that your child is given, just do whatever you can to get the services and help that you and your child need.
- The future is scary. Plan for it, but do not dwell in its uncertainty. It is often easier to take things day-by-day or moment-by-moment.
- Forgive yourself for sacrificing daily chores (i.e., dusting and vacuuming) for quality time spent with loved ones, as well as for time for yourself. I have learned the hard way, that if I do not take time for myself (whether it is to pamper myself, relax, or go out with friends), I cannot be the best that I need to be for my family.
- Hook up with other parents. They are a tremendous amount of support and information.
- Explore all of your treatment options, but remember to be skeptical and weigh the benefits and the risks. Whatever you decide, you are the one who has to deal with the feelings like. 'if only I had tried this or not done this...'
- Be consistent and deal with problem behaviors when your children are little (they will not be cute or easy to handle when your child is bigger).
- Take time to educate others.
- Remember, you can do more than you think you can, and you probably already are.
- Celebrate and appreciate all successes, no matter how big or small.

"I am blessed to have family and friends who support us both emotionally and by lending a helping hand."

Lana, Robbie & Harrison

Maryland

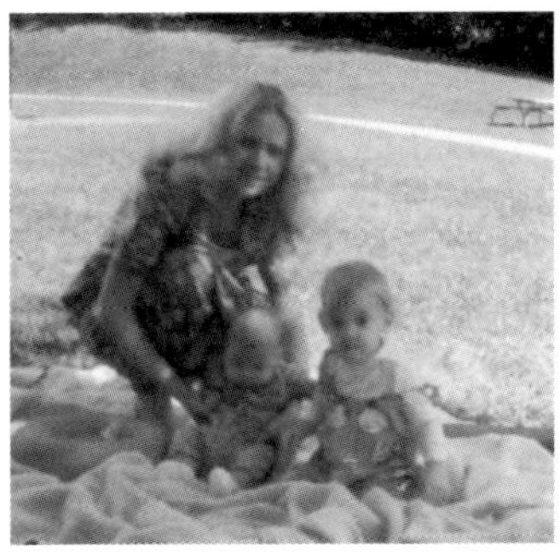

Robbie was diagnosed at 4 years
Harrison was diagnosed at 3 years

CONTACT:
tunick42004@yahoo.com

BIGGEST CHALLENGE(S)

My biggest challenge has been communication with Harrison who is non-verbal. He never picked up on sign language or pointing. He takes my hand when he wants something. We are starting to use augmentive devices. Toilet training has also been a very great challenge.

GREATEST BLESSING(S)

My greatest blessing has been the birth of both my children. I thank God for having them as they are both very precious to me.

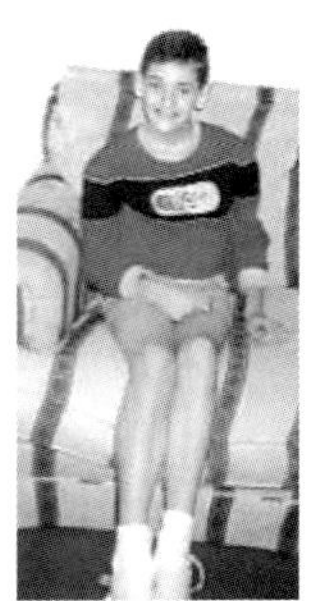

WORDS OF WISDOM

Look at the bright side of what your children can do and then work from there. Have patience and live it day by day.

LaShell & Aaron

Wisconsin

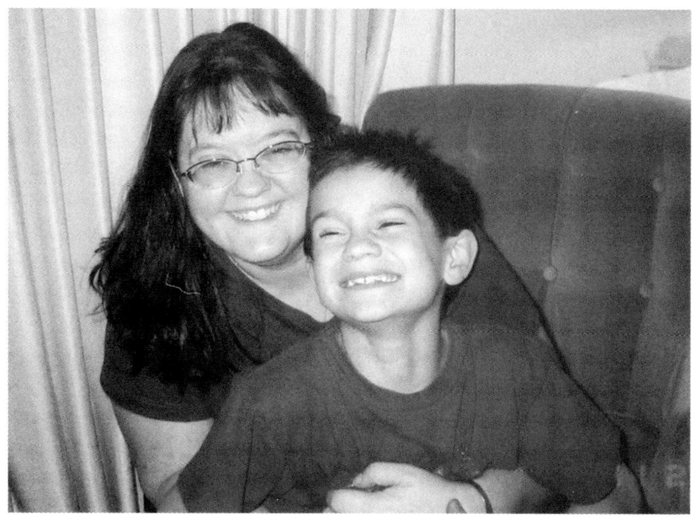

CONTACT:
Rothfelder@aol.com

Aaron was diagnosed at 9 years

BIGGEST CHALLENGE(S)

While there have been many challenges thus far, the biggest two have been finding services and facing my own fears and feelings. Services have been very difficult to find due to his not being diagnosed with Asperger's Syndrome until age nine. I took him to many doctors and therapists. I have known "something" wasn't right since he was two or three years old. No one would give me a firm answer regarding Aaron. Everyone (until the Asperger's specialist finally diagnosed him) had said, "Well, he's borderline" this and that or, "He just doesn't fit any one diagnosis and it is not autism because he looked at me." Well, this was in an "ideal" one-to-one assessment, yet school kept sending notes home with, "he is causing trouble for himself. He's invading other's space. He won't pay attention." Finally, a few weeks after his ninth birthday, I took him to an Asperger's specialist who diagnosed him. I thought, "Finally, I can get him the help he deserves." I was wrong. He did not qualify for treatment for autism through the Medicaid Waiver program because he was "too old." He had to have started a program by the time he turned eight. We were one year and three weeks too late. I did finally apply and was approved for the family support program for Aaron. This in no way comes close to providing the help Aaron would have received had he been diagnosed earlier, but at least it is something. We are going to try hippotherapy (therapeutic horseback riding.) I will also be able to get him into summer camp this summer.

Facing my own fears and guilt has also been very difficult. Many questions have gone through my head, "What will Aaron's life be like? Will he ever be "normal"? Will he ever have friends? Will he hold a job, date, get married or be happy?" I have cried many nights wondering, worrying and feeling guilty. I felt that I should have done something different and Aaron would not have Asperger's. I have since come to understand and accept that he has it and it was NOT my fault. It is difficult when you have a child, who appears "normal and healthy" and then some time later, is diagnosed with an autism spectrum disorder. The most important thing is to recognize the strengths (in your child, yourself and those who support you) and build on them.

Greatest Blessings

I will forever be thankful for the many strangers who have believed in Aaron and have helped him. They have given us hope for his future. It is truly wonderful to see Aaron's face light up when he sees them.

Aaron, himself, is also a blessing. He always goes to each appointment with a smile. He loves animals and being outside in nature and wants to be a vet when he grows up. Music is therapeutic for him and he loves to listen and even played violin for awhile. He is so sweet and caring and my beautiful boy. He is truly a blessing to me, his dad, his brother and sister and all who know him.

Words of Wisdom

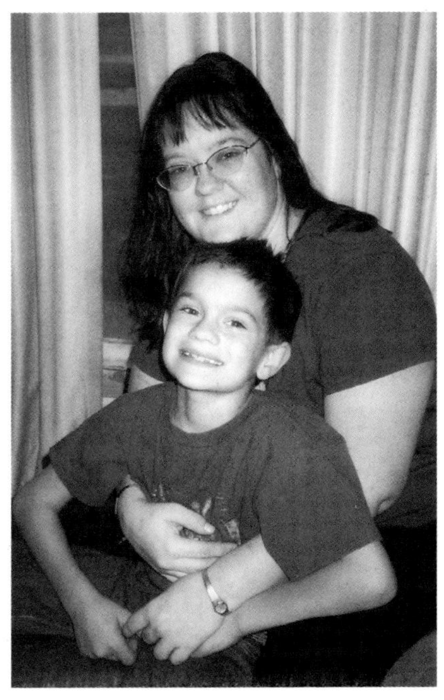

"Never give up!" Aaron has taught me this through his persistence and smile at every appointment he has and every obstacle he hurdles. He hasn't given up despite his challenges. He is my son and no matter what, I will never give up on him. He loves to hear this and to know that Mom is there always.

"As a Mother, you know your child best. Go with your instincts." I felt something wasn't right. I would believe that Aaron was "bad" or "doing this on purpose." This goes along with never giving up. You know your child. Fight for what is best for him/her.

"Take time for yourself." It is important for us to care for ourselves in order to care for our children. If we are so worn out we can't care for ourselves, how would we be able to take care of our children?

Laura & Hunter

Indiana

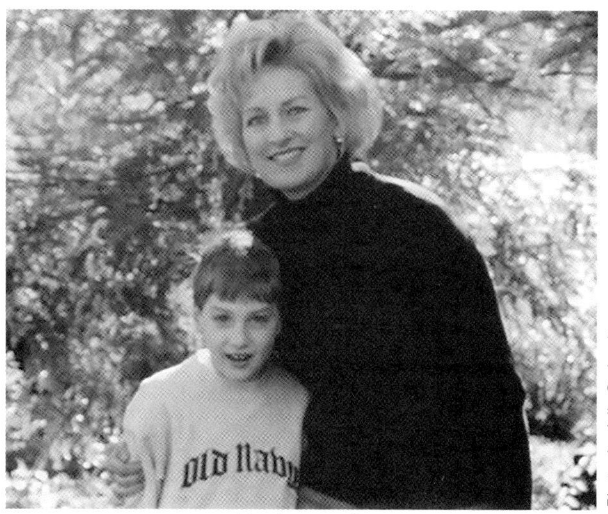

Photos by Julie Gerhardt

Hunter age 9

CONTACT:
LMccord@ecommunity.com

Hunter was diagnosed at 3 years

BIGGEST CHALLENGE(S)

Emotional challenge: Not knowing what Hunter's future will be when I am no longer here for him. Will he have to live a lonely life in a world where nothing makes sense to him and no one will appreciate him or love him or hug him or kiss him? I can barely stand the thought of him without me.

Physical challenge: Behavior problems at home and in public…"screaming", "throwing objects", "self-injuring". I try to always remember that there is a little boy locked in this illness-stricken body just trying to communicate and be understood. It's not all good, but neither is having a "normal" child…I'm raising a 17 year old daughter also and I can tell you that it's just as challenging!

Greatest Blessings

Having the support of family and friends. Having a place of employment that has been willingly flexible. There are rewards with the struggle...know how strong you can be and how much you can love. Hunter was sent to inspire me. Hunter's compassion makes me glow, when he's sweet, he's sincere to the core. What is more terrifying than living with his illness is the thought of living without him.

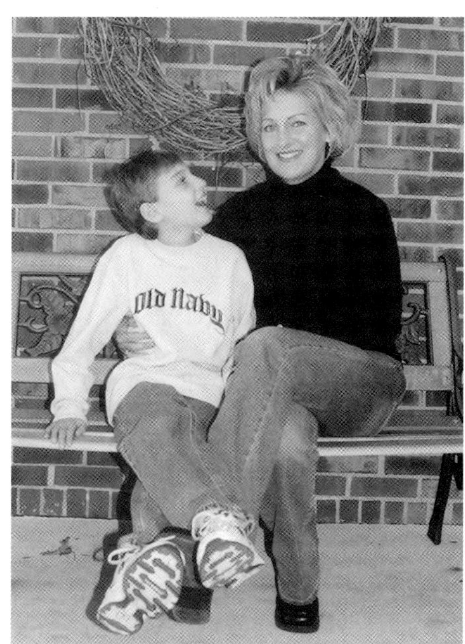

Words of Wisdom

Contact your nearest early intervention program and ask to be put on the autism waiver list. There is a waiting list and the sooner you get put on it, the better. My son has been on the waiting list since he was 3 years old and he's now 9 and still waiting! The waiver program offers all types of therapy and financial assistance without the parent's income taken into consideration.

You will never get over it, but you will adapt and connect in a special way unlike any other. There is a bond that is indescribable.

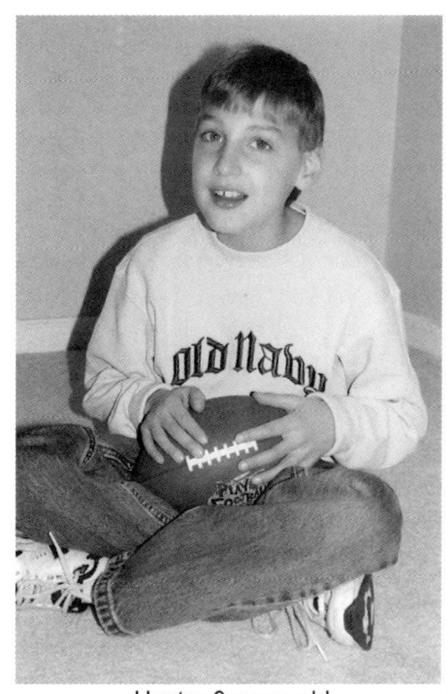

Hunter 9 years old

"You will never get over it, but you will adapt and connect in a special way unlike any other. There is a bond that is indescribable."

Laura & Phillip

Texas

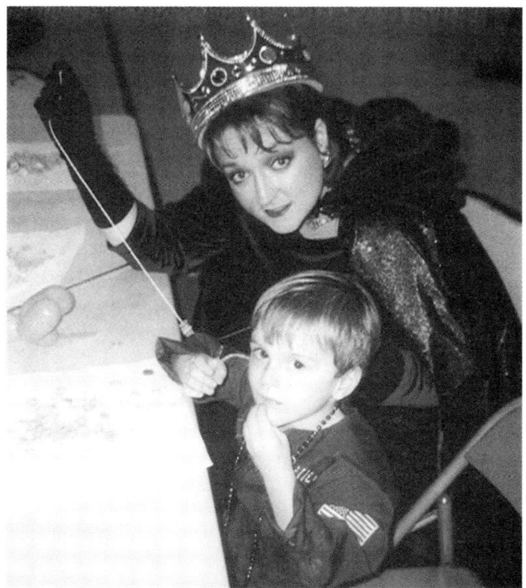

CONTACT:
www.marykay.com//santos

Phillip was diagnosed at 4 years

Recovery from Autism is Possible

As I lie in my bedroom on my comfy bed, looking through lace curtains into a green tropical backyard on an overcast, but not quite cloudy day, thoughts race through my head. What in the world did I do to deserve a load like this? Can God actually expect me to be the mother of an autistic child? Can he expect me to be a good Christian servant, wife, mother of two (one autistic), business owner and crusader for children with autism?

The answer comes, "Yep."

Through my tears I search my soul for that secret reservoir of strength that God seems to have reserved for and honored only women with.

The answer comes, "You are a good Christian Servant, wife, mother of 2 (one autistic), business owner, and I chose you to be a crusader for children with autism because of who you are. You are a woman and … I made you of stronger stuff."

2 Timothy 1:7
"For God did not give us the spirit of timidity, but a spirit of power, of love and self-discipline."

So, what do I do every day? I wake up and thank God for my blessings—especially for the blessing of a child with autism. You see, my son is on the DAN! (Defeat Autism Now!) Protocol. Every day, we recover something new. Every day I thank God humbly for sending me on the path to recovery and for my DAN! doctor. Every day I watch Phillip (my autistic son) do something new that autistic kids aren't supposed to do.

Then comes the thought – What did I do to deserve to be blessed like this—watching the awakening of a stolen mind? What an honor!

Favorite Resources:

1) www.autsimresearchinstitute.com to order the DAN! Protocol and find a DAN! Doctor in your area www.doctorvolpe.com
2) *Unraveling the Mystery of Autism and PDD*, by Karen Seroussi

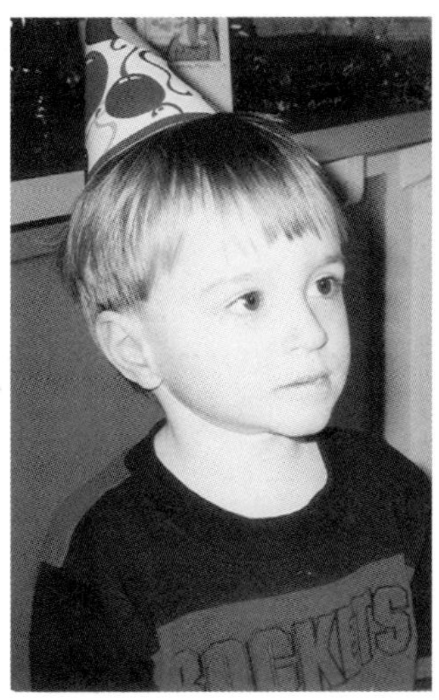

Phillip disappears age 3½

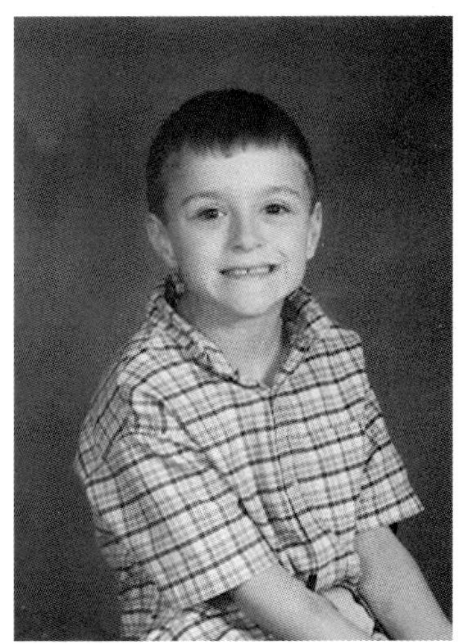

Phillip today

Laurie & James

Indiana

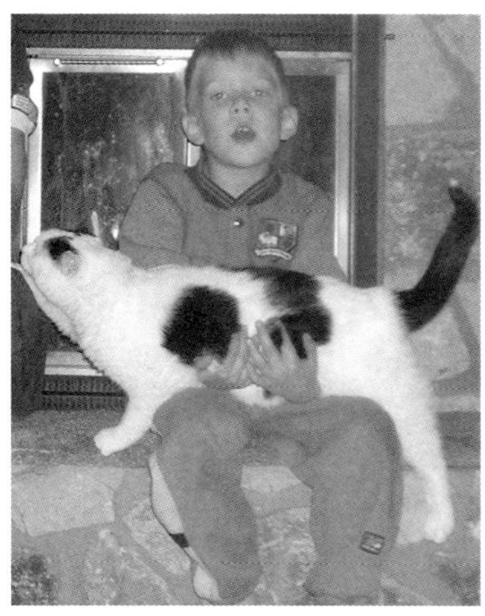

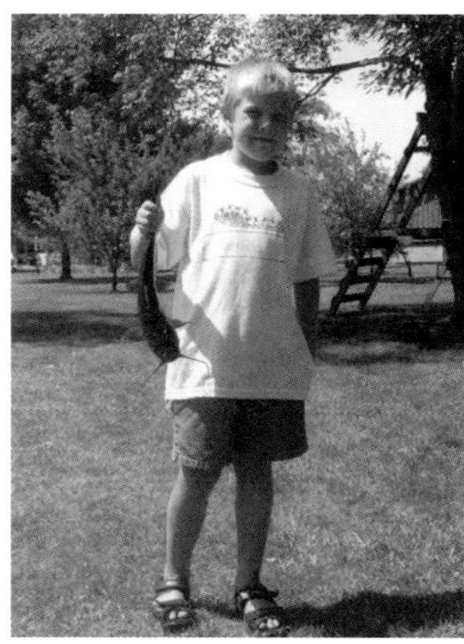

James age 8

CONTACT:

LJCallahan@Ameritech.Net

James was diagnosed PDD-NOS at 5 years

BIGGEST CHALLENGE(S)

After I recovered from my own denial of the problem, my biggest challenge in helping James was dealing with friends and family members. At first, they were saying that "maybe" something was wrong. But, after we got a diagnosis, they insisted that he couldn't possibly have PDD (pervasive developmental disorder). When I started pursuing alternative therapies to treat his condition, the people who were closest to me insisted that the therapy was causing his problems instead of treating them.

One of the first things we tried was putting him on a special diet. I was very quickly convinced that a special diet was a big piece of the puzzle when I saw dramatic improvement in the first few weeks. Unfortunately, James couldn't have cookies, bread, milk, candy, Kool-Aid, or anything else that other preschoolers ate. People said, "Of course he acts so crazy – you aren't letting him be a little boy! Just give him a cookie once in awhile so he can be like everybody else!" At this point in his treatment, I was completely alone. Nobody understood. Nobody wanted to understand. Everybody just wanted somebody to blame, and who better to blame than "the refrigerator mom". Blaming the mother's parenting style for a child's disabilities has been a tradition for many years. And why not? It is a conveniently simple explanation that is difficult to refute.

Since the diet was only one of many pieces to my son's puzzle, people didn't see that it was helping until a few years later. After 3 years of being very strict with his diet, trying every non-invasive therapy I could find, and pouring my entire life into helping my son, he started to show improvement. People started noticing that he was getting better. Then they suggested that maybe nothing was ever wrong in the first place. Maybe he is just outgrowing this mysterious behavior. Does he really need to be on that crazy diet? Then, we slip up and accidentally give him some trace amount of food that is "illegal" for him. He has a violent reaction that nobody can deny, and finally they are convinced. At least for now.

Today, I get a little more respect from family members about the therapies. A few people have even tried some of the same things for themselves and been successful. When he grows up, I hope that James can get more respect from people as an adult who has recovered from a "hopeless" condition. Maybe if he really does become a doctor, he will have enough credibility for people to believe him.

Greatest Blessings

Our greatest blessing from our experiences has been that we are much more humble than we would have been without them. Since our children are on a very restricted diet, they don't even want all the candy, carbonated drinks, cake, potato chips, etc. that most children seem to live on. We spend so much time and money on therapy that we have never had video games, fancy clothes, or expensive toys. It seems that many children seem to live for the current fad. My boys usually don't care to follow the crowd. Since following the crowd has never been an option for them, they don't feel the pressure to conform that other kids feel.

James is proud to wear clothes that were handed down from other families, and he proudly eats grapes or an apple for a snack while the other kids eat pre-packaged snack foods. Sometimes, when the other kids comment on his "weird" food, he gives them a short lecture on nutrition. His feelings are not hurt, and he knows that his food is better for his body than the junk food that most people eat. At the age if 8, he has already learned that following the crowd is usually not the best way to go.

He also has great empathy for other children with disabilities. When he sees somebody who has any kind of disability, he reaches out to them. Even when he meets a person who is so severely disabled that they don't seem to be aware of his presence, he talks to them just like he would talk to anybody else. Instead of looking away in embarrassment, he treats them the same way he would treat anybody else. I always hope that for a few moments his new friend can forget that they are different because a little boy speaks to them as if the disability doesn't exist.

> "Nobody understood. Nobody wanted to understand. Everybody just wanted somebody to blame, and who better to blame than 'the refrigerator mom'".

Words of Wisdom

When James was 5 years old, a psychologist broke the news to us that he had some form of autism. She said that he would never really grow up, he would never have friends, and that we should never expect him to be able to do the things that other kids his age do. He just won't understand. She also advised us not to spend lots of time and money trying to help him because it would never accomplish anything. She said that we should enjoy him while he was young but be prepared to institutionalize him by the time he was a teenager. I guess in a way, her prognosis made sense. He didn't understand pretend play, he couldn't answer even the simplest questions, and his only speech was this monotonous monologue that meant almost nothing to other people.

Instead of following her advice, I took it as a threat. That would be his future if I didn't do anything to help him. So, that's when I started reading every autism book I could get my hands on. First, I discovered the special diet, then mercury poisoning, yeast overgrowth, and sensory integration dysfunction. That was just in the first year. I treated every piece as I discovered it even though the world was against me. I had doctors tell me that I was wasting my time, and I had family members tell me that I was causing all of his trouble by torturing him with my ridiculous ideas. People accused me of child abuse, child neglect, and being overprotective. In that first year of treatment, I think I heard every kind of unwanted advice and accusation imaginable.

In the past year or so, people have started noticing that James is doing much better. He no longer has mercury poisoning, he has friends, he is on grade-level (with some special help), he does understand most things that boys his age understand, and he is growing up. If the psychologist who saw him 3 years ago met him today, she wouldn't recognize him. We have never even considered putting him in an institution. He is still struggling with Bipolar Disorder, he has some learning problems, and he is still on that "crazy" diet, but he does have a pretty good chance at life now. We have come a long way in 3 years, and we still have a long way to go. We just have to keep up the pace. He tells me that when he grows up, he wants to become a doctor who will cure autism for free. That is the goal that I am shooting for. My job is to do everything I can to give him that potential.

When I meet parents who have recently gotten a diagnosis of PDD for their child, I share my experiences with them. I tell them how hard is has been, and I always emphasize that we can NEVER GIVE UP on our children. Even when the whole world seems to be against us, we have to keep going. As soon as we give up, there is not much hope. It takes lots of work to cure a condition like PDD. It would also be nice if more people had support from family and friends. The treatments might be more successful if the parents didn't feel like they were alone in the world trying to treat a hopeless condition.

I hope this book can provide some of the support that parents need to help cure their children.

Linda & Mike

Connecticut

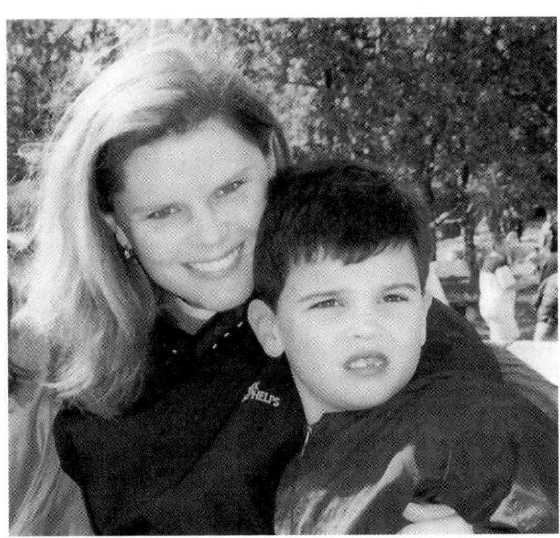

CONTACT:
LMDENNING@comcast.net

Mike was diagnosed at 3 years

BIGGEST CHALLENGE(S)

My son Michael's autism diagnosis cast a gray cloud over our family. My husband cashed out emotionally as if Mike's issues were a personal failure he needed to reconcile. Our inability to communicate effectively about our loss was a huge factor in the breakdown of our 7-year marriage. As the primary caretaker for my children, there was nothing left to do but "suck it up" and make a mission to make sense of it all, which was (and continues to be even today!) no small feat.

My daughter Sarah was 5 years old when we divorced. She had a difficult time understandably; not only feeling the loss of having a brother 14 months her junior that she couldn't really relate to, but watching her Dad build a home and a life across town as well. Sarah and I continue to have the same conversations, even today, 7 years later... "Why aren't you and Dad together anymore?" and, "Why do you have to help Michael with everything when you expect me to take care of myself?" My responses have gotten more complex over the years, but the facts remain... her Dad couldn't handle it, and her brother is still autistic. Without a crystal ball there's no way to know if either of those things would improve over time.

As is true for many people with autism, my son has many severe sensory deficiencies. Potty training, haircuts and dental visits were nothing short of wrestling matches and mixed tears with Mike and I for many years. I was told by many parents that these "learning opportunities" would get better with time and to never give up. Today, Mike is independent in the bathroom, proudly opens his mouth for the dentist and always greets our hairdresser Darlene with a big smile and hug. Mike has gone from only eating toast with peanut butter, applesauce and oodles of goldfish crackers to sitting down in a restaurant ordering his own meals of hamburgers, chicken and pizza. For us, the little victories are celebrated as exuberantly as the major childhood milestones.

My challenge today lies in the ambiguity of Michael's future. I lay awake at night wondering about many things… 'will puberty derail the excellent progress we're making?... Will Mike ever be able to have a job or live away from home when he's older?' Most of my concerns lie around what will ultimately happen once I die. Who will take up the reins and be his advocate? And, there's the whole estate planning issue that I have yet to be brave enough to tackle.

Greatest Blessings

First and foremost, Mike sleeps like a champ! It seems as if he knows that his Mom needs at least 7 hours of sleep to function… it's his daily gift to me.

For all of Michael's unique quirks, he has a wonderful sense of humor and enthusiasm for life. He's advanced enough in his sophistication to understand many things, but not too advanced to even care about the things that cause worry for many of us "typical" folks. What an enviable place to be! He is in a protected world where his biggest concern is finding his favorite video jacket when it's fallen behind the bed. Mike capably participates in many of the same activities enjoyed by his typical peers, like trips to the local library, swimming and horseback riding. We live in a town where the schools truly have Mike's best interest at heart. I cannot imagine the anguish of other families who have to fight for appropriate services or are not treated as equals in their child's educational process. We are very fortunate and I do not take this for granted.

Last and most important, the key people in Michael's life are truly our greatest blessings. I wouldn't have made it through the divorce and aftermath without my parents and our amazing childcare provider Emogene. My fiancé John has stepped up to the plate as my partner and daily support system for Mike. Sarah has proven Mike's best teacher of all. We are truly blessed by her patience and eagerness to see him succeed.

Words of Wisdom

By design it's hard for any Mom to put herself first, let alone one with a child with special needs — but it's essential that you build in a little "selfish Mommy" time into your busy schedule once in a while…. take a bubble bath, go to the gym, have Grandma come over so you can enjoy an evening out with your husband or girlfriends. You will be better equipped to meet your family's needs when you are happy, rested and emotionally centered. Also, VOLUNTEER! Not only is it a rewarding way to give back to a supportive community, but it helps to put your own family's situation in perspective by sharing struggles with other special needs families.

Finally, I've learned that it's not a sign of weakness to ask for help when you truly need it. The only way I have kept my sanity to see my son's 11th birthday is by accepting the generosity of my family and closest friends. I thank God for them every day.

One other pearl of wisdom I would like to share with newly-diagnosed families... when nosy but well-meaning people approach you in the grocery store with scrutiny about your inability to control your child's unacceptable behavior, take a deep breath and say, "I'm glad you cared enough to ask... my son has autism, and his outbursts are because he has difficulty communicating his wants and needs..." Not only will it show that you ARE truly in control, but you will broaden their horizons as well. Speaking for myself, it has been very difficult over the years defending Mike's behaviors against public (mis)perception. Mike, like other kids with autism, bears no tell-tale sign of a disability on his forehead. Over the years I have found that most people are genuinely curious about our kids and don't really mean to be rude or inappropriate. However, if they are intolerant, it's ultimately THEIR problem, not ours.

If your experience is like mine, you're asked quite often, "How do you do it?" My immediate reaction is, "I just do... I've known no other way." When it comes down to it, we love our kids unconditionally, warts and all. We persevere every day to make life better for them... we just do. There IS no other way.

Favorite Resources:

1) *One Small Starfish: A Mother's Everyday Advice, Survival Tactics and Wisdom for Raising a Special Needs Child* by Anne Addison
2) *Behavioral Interventions for Young Children with Autism*, edited by Catherine Maurice
3) *Siblings of Autism: A Guide for Families* by Sandra L. Harris, Ph.D
4) *Children with Autism: A Parent's Guide* edited by Michael D. Powers, Psy.D
5) www.autism-society.org
6) www.canfoundation.org
7) www.autism-resources.com
8) www.wrightslaw.com
9) www.autism-pdd.net
10) www.AutismResearchInstitute.com
11) www.autism.org
12) www.autism-ally.com
13) www.ctfeat.org
14) www.equistrides.org

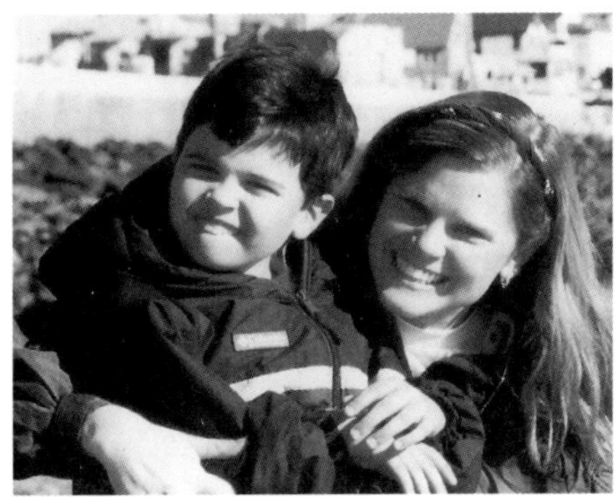

LeAnne & Alex

Wisconsin

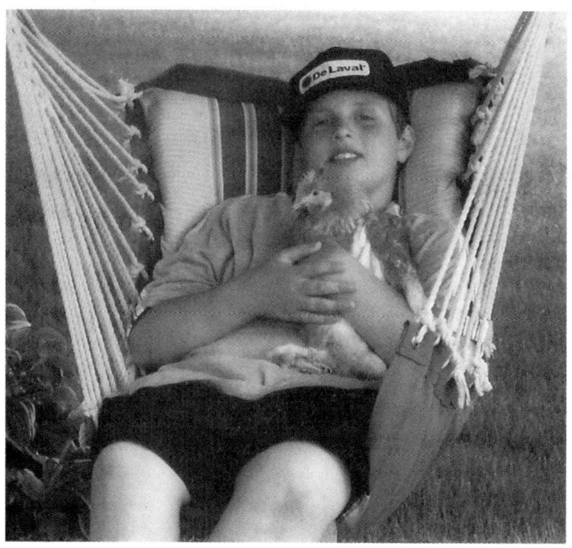

CONTACT:
nlmlsna@centurytel.net

Alex was diagnosed at 2½ years

BIGGEST CHALLENGE(S)

One of the biggest challenges I have found raising our son Alex is the helplessness I sometimes feel. I love our son so much and I, of course want him to be happy and healthy. I have always strived to find the best treatment for him. Because of his chronic allergies it is sometimes hard to know what the true issues are with his behavior.

It can be very costly as well as emotionally draining with all of the 'so-called' cures and treatments for autism. We, as parents, are very vulnerable and will do almost anything to help our children.

Greatest Blessings

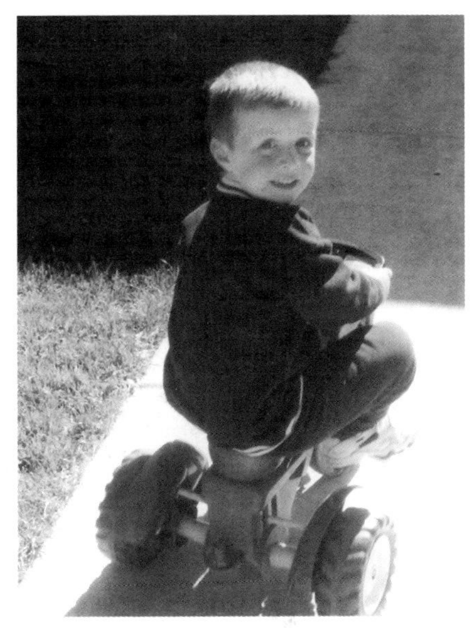

When Alex was about 3 years old, I finally realized just what a blessing he truly was to our lives. I learned very quickly that raising a child with autism can be very daunting. I also realized that God only picks those of us that can truly "handle" the responsibility. When I first found out about the autism I was so scared and angry. But today I thank God for giving Alex to us. He is a wonderful young boy who is growing into a fine young man. Alex has a true connection with the Lord and he is helping all of us see life in a new way. Alex has so much to share. We, as a family, have met so many wonderful people in the autism community. Alex has touched so many lives in his short 10½ years. He has left a spot in so many people's hearts. It is amazing to watch as he learned the most simple things we all take for granted. I remember when he was about 5 and he came to me with a dandelion and said, "Here mom, I love you." I still have that dandelion and I remember how I thought I would never hear those words. To me, that is a blessing I will never forget.

Words of Wisdom

PATIENCE

This is the single most important thing we as parents need to learn. I remember when I was pregnant with Alex. I was on bed rest and I was in the hospital for 2 weeks before I delivered him at 35 weeks. I was so restless and hated lying still. I had a nurse that told me everyday, "Be patient. Every day that he has inside his chances are better for a healthier start." I remember telling her the one thing I didn't have was patience. She said, "You will learn." She was right and that is what we need most of all. Patience!! These little people need us to watch over them and admire the small things they accomplish. They will do most of it, it will just be a little later then most. Marvel in the wonder of who they really are. Love them for what they have learned. God knew that I needed to learn patience that is why he gave Alex to me. I thank him everyday for that.

> "Marvel in the wonder of who they really are. Love them for what they have learned".

Linda & William

Wisconsin

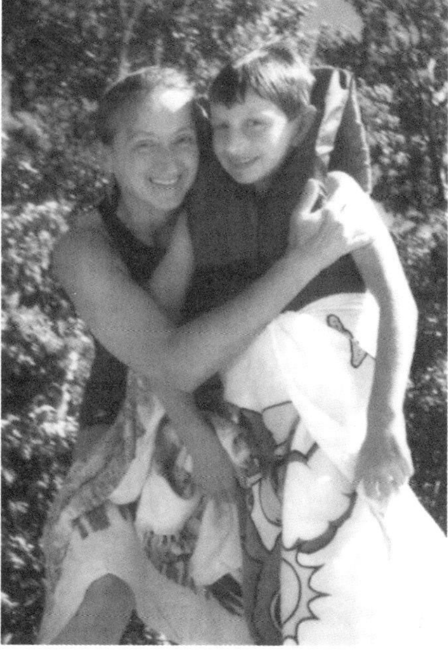

William is 13 years old

CONTACT:
ltollefs@uwc.edu

William was diagnosed at 3 years

BIGGEST CHALLENGE(S)

Hard to say. The challenges are different with every developmental period. The most difficult so far has been two aggressive periods — one at age 6 and another at age 12-13. Another constant challenge is to negotiate the tension between pushing him too much (so he's frustrated) and not pushing him hard enough (doing too much for him).

GREATEST BLESSINGS

Other families with autistic members are a tremendous source of wisdom, support, and humor. Also, our kids really push us to develop our inner resources — patience, compassion, intuition, assertiveness, critical thinking, and empathy.

WORDS OF WISDOM

Don't be too hard on yourself. When I become self-critical about all that is not getting done, or not getting done well, I repeat this mantra: "I'm doing the best I can with the time and the resources I have available."

Taking Care

by Linda Tollefsrud

My child isn't talking, plays alone, lines up toy trains.
A lifetime of labels (autism? PDD? OCD?) starts its turning.
The doctors, not knowing what else to say,
not knowing how to help, urging:
Remember to take care of yourself.

The race is on, running from behavior therapy to vitamins,
pursuing cutting edge treatments and miracle cures,
hour after hour, dollar after dollar.
Sleepless nights after anxious days:
Remember to take care of yourself.

Scanning the brain,
counting calories and nutrients,
analyzing blood, urine, DNA; you-name-it-I'll-try-it,
(scurrying to that 'other' full-time job!)
Remember to take care of yourself.

Whirlwind trips conferring and connecting,
gurus of drugs and diet dissecting this "case,"
friendships spun within a worldwide web,
the latest research cavorting through dreams:
Remember to take care of yourself.

Weaving a secure net of support
From the bare threads of programs, placement, respite
and the thin air of transition and adult services,
Tying the knots with whispers and heartstrings:
Remember to take care of yourself.

Lazing the weekend away,
a kettle of soup slowly simmering on the stove,
walking the dogs through the woods,
making love leisurely and often:
It's a fantasy, but it sustains me.

In the glare of reality, I know
this merry-go-round is so much a part of me,
if it stopped, I would be
forever reeling.
Remember. Take care, yourself.

Lisa & Arrian

Georgia

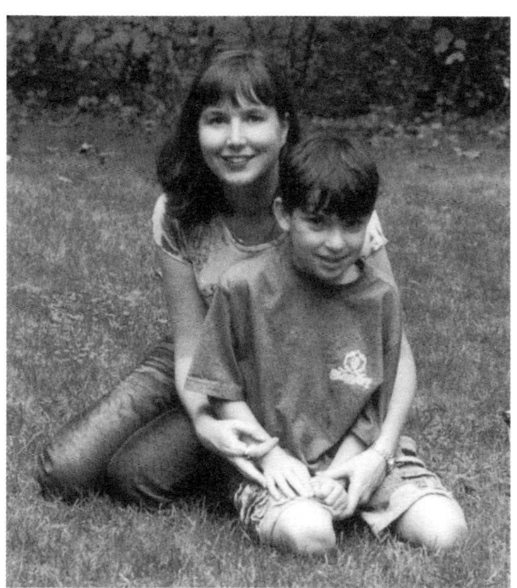

Arrian, 7 years old, 2004

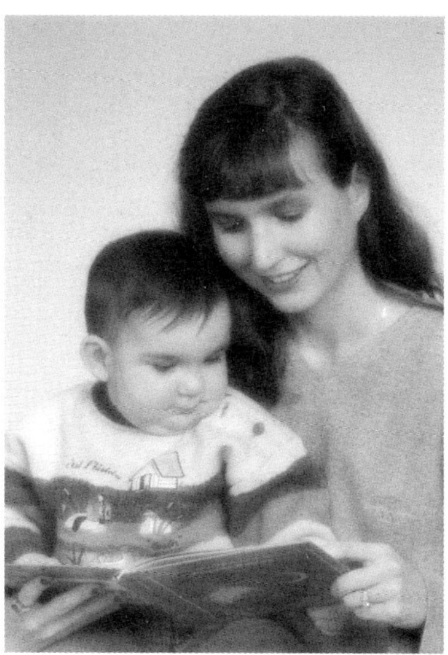

Arrian 11 months old

Arrian was diagnosed at 5 years

BIGGEST CHALLENGE(S)

The biggest challenge I have is knowing that biomedical and behavior treatment is out there, but figuring out how to achieve getting it. The cost is astronomical. It is hard for outsiders to understand that autism is treatable and the treatment plan is one that insurance companies do not want to help with. It is a constant battle to get the services my son needs, but one I fight every day.

GREATEST BLESSINGS

The greatest blessing is my son! He is the love of my life. He is a trooper and a fighter. With all his hardships, he enters the world every day with a smile on his face, ready to conquer the world.

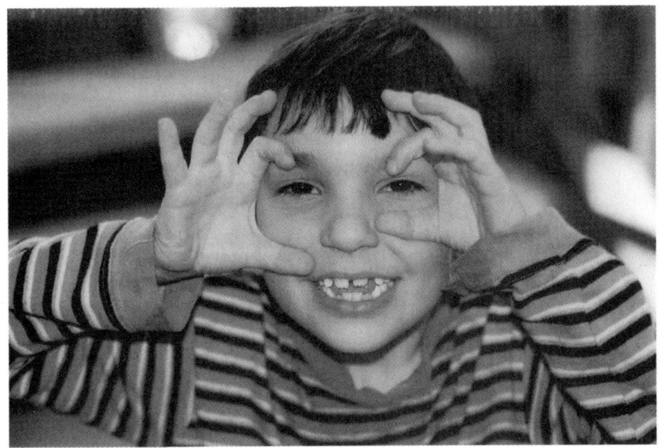

Arrian imitating "cheese, take a picture!" Age 6

Words of Wisdom

Don't be judgmental. Be careful what you say. My all-time favorite line from a dear friend is, "Oh, I thought he wasn't talking because you never talked to him." If you see a mother at the grocery store and her child is out of control, do not go to her and tell her all the child needs is a good spanking! One of my favorite quotes, but I don't remember who originally said it, is "If spanking could cure my child, believe me, I would be more than happy to spank him." Lots of autistic children look like their typical peers.

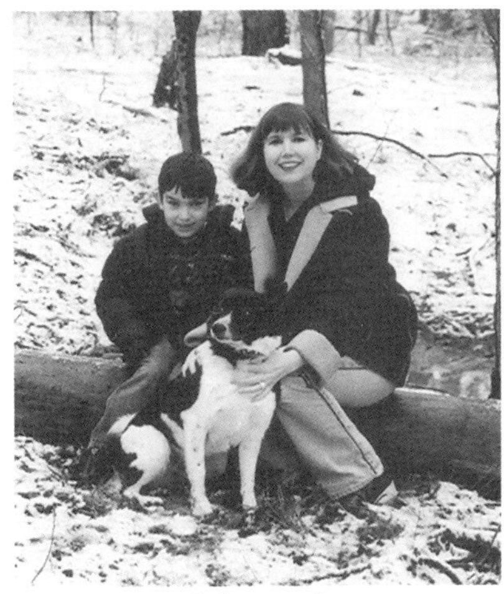

Arrian age 6

Lori & Samantha

Minnesota

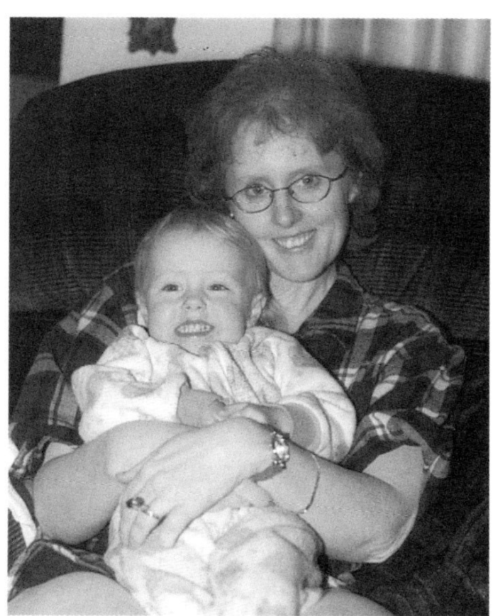

CONTACT:
twandlw@mnns.com

Samantha was diagnosed at 4 years

BIGGEST CHALLENGE(S)

The bomb was dropped on November 11, 2002. I will never forget the date. It is etched in my mind as securely as any birth date or anniversary. The day my beautiful 4-year-old girl was diagnosed as autistic. Since then I have faced many challenges as a mother. The biggest of these include:

- Finding and holding on to hope for her future. A mother must have hope. At times this is difficult, but I always look for bright things in our lives. Samantha's love for music, her ability to sing songs even though she cannot speak to me, her laugh, the bright sparkle in her eyes when she looks at me. All these things give me hope.
- Finding the strength to continue to work on communication. The loss of Samantha's verbal language at age two was the hardest thing to adjust to. Now the only time I am able to hear my baby's voice is when she is under stress and calling for me to help her. This is a tremendous challenge to remain strong and hopeful that someday we can talk to each other in more loving situations.

- The loss of verbal language has also caused the challenge of not knowing what Samantha needs, not understanding when she is sick and in pain. She is unable to tell me what is wrong, where it hurts, or how she feels. This is the stuff of mother's nightmares, and the biggest challenge to try to deal with and learn to overcome.

Greatest Blessings

I have been granted many blessings that I must not lose sight of:

- I have a beautiful, happy child who loves me.
- I have a wonderful happy and healthy son, who loves his big sister and helps out by teaching her how to play together.
- Even though we live in a very rural area, we have wonderful public education and in-home therapy available that is helping Samantha improve her quality of life through education and treatment. I was blessed to find other parents of autistic children who shared my pain and we learned to support and encourage each other. This is a vital lifeline for me.

Words of Wisdom

If I were to give another parent of an autistic child any words of wisdom, I would say:

- Go ahead and cry for a while. This is a devastating thing at first and it is OK to let your feelings out. Then try to focus on those challenges before you and find the strength to tackle them.
- Get your child enrolled in educational and therapeutic services and yourself involved in a parent support group as soon as possible. Don't wait.
- Do your best to not let the insensitivity of others get to you. Once I was working at an autism awareness conference and I had a mother tell me, "Thank God my children are OK." I found this rather insensitive and it upset me at first, but then I tried to tell myself that this is exactly why we need more autism awareness, for people like her.
- Do what you need to do for yourself. For me, I found getting involved and advocating for better laws and services helped me feel like I was doing something. But this is not the path for all mothers. Find what makes you feel good about yourself and your family, and do it.

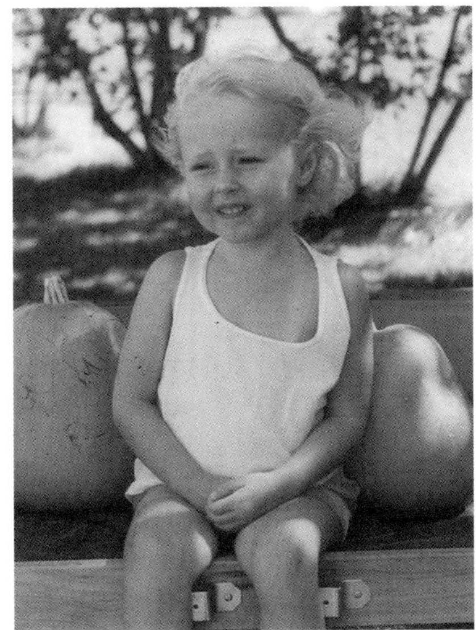

My Samantha is now a 6-year-old kindergartner and loving school. I take pleasure in her love of school. We never know what is in store for any of our children. We can only do the best we can and pray for their safety and happiness.

Luanne & Tre'

Canada

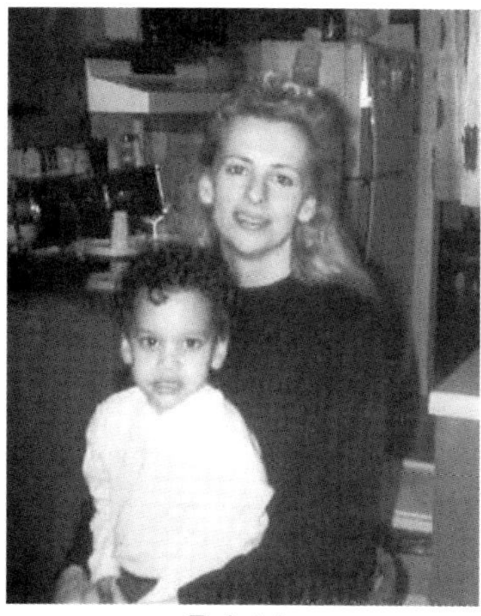

Tre' at 4

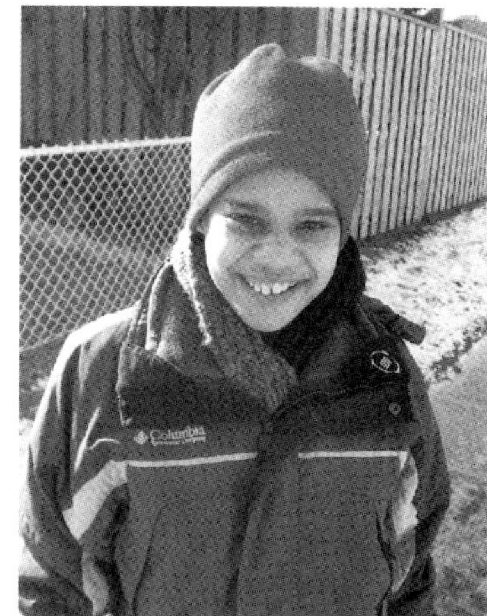

Tre' age 12, 2005

CONTACT:
kinda379@yahoo.com

Tre' was diagnosed at 3½ years

BIGGEST CHALLENGE(S)

Imagine for a moment that you are unable to understand the words people speak or what the movements mean in Sign Language or what simple picture symbols are trying to say or explain. Now take one more step and realize that you are also unable to speak, to form language, and you will see how my son Tre' lives, thinks and feels.

My son is a beautiful 12-year-old boy with big almond eyes, curly brown hair and dimples. To the casual observer, he appears to be like any other child, that is, until you take a few minutes to observe him. It is then that you will realize that he is different and it will also be noticed that he has a raised and bruised bump in the middle of his forehead, put there by years of head banging against any hard or sharp surface. He has a specially made blue helmet made of space-age material that will not break. It is utilized when he begins a tantrum, yet he still gets in a few bangs before it can be put on. Tre' no longer lives with me but lives in a group residence with 7 other children with various disabilities and trained staff who can deal with him and teach him with constant supervision. He is a biter, but his self-injurious behaviors are more prominent. He has been in this residence since he was 7½ and I miss him every single day. I felt I had no choice but to finally accept the help that was offered to me as he was growing bigger and stronger and was beginning to bite me as well. I was alone in raising him and worn out and this was the safest move for both of us. Without the help I received from DLC (the residence) and its owner and incredible staff, I don't know if we would be here today, in one piece anyway.

Greatest Blessings

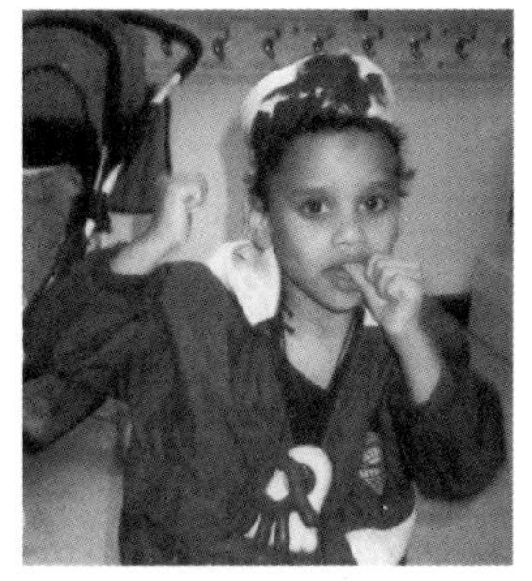

I see other parents of special needs children with their struggles and know that I was incredibly blessed, not only for the help I received but the numerous people and agencies and workers that all took a special interest in my beautiful boy and I. The caliber of people involved over the years was unbelievable in its depth — the behavior analysts, nurses, social workers, doctors, and psychologists. I had incredible workers that spent 2 hours a day, 5 days a week for over 4 years performing Intensive Behavior Intervention Therapy. Students working through the university in areas of psychology and teaching (and sometimes not) were all incredibly dedicated to helping Tre'. I can't begin to thank them all.

It was Tre' though, that blessed me most of all. Through him, and him alone, he made me a better person. He made me look outside my own concerns and myself, he made me see what was really important and made me see people and things in a different light. I became his biggest advocate, fiercely fighting for what he deserved from school boards, daycares, doctors, government services and society at large. He gave me passion and anyone knows that a mother's love is the strongest tool you can have behind you.

Words of Wisdom

I used to be a quiet person, unwilling to bring attention to myself, content in the background of life. I no longer had that choice or luxury if I was to help my son. I am sure, in retrospect, that many schools and agencies cringed when they saw me, knowing I was there, once again, advocating for Tre' one more time. Tre' has no voice, I had to speak for both of us, if I didn't he was lost and that was not an option. There is no time for heartbreaking depression or paralyzing grief. It is vitally important that the mourning for 'what could have been' is quickly embraced, the loss acknowledged then set aside. You must work with what you have, make the best choices for 'what is' and move forward with a stoic mindset to find the very best you are able to get for your child. Taking too much time in denial, or endlessly searching for all the reasons why your child is the way they are, is a monumental loss of time better spent on getting the best services and therapies available for your child.

For those of you that are living this very special life with your unique child, your strength and tenacity is vital to your child. Never give up! Never accept "This is the way we've always done it" when you suggest a better more effective way of teaching him or her. Never accept inferior services so as not to 'rock the boat'; and finally, love your child for who they are not for what you previously wished for them to be. They are perfectly them and they are here to teach us, to teach society, that being different is their destiny and it is us who are blessed to have been chosen to share in their lives.

> "He gave me passion and anyone knows that a mother's love is the strongest tool you can have behind you."

Lynda & Rohr

Washington

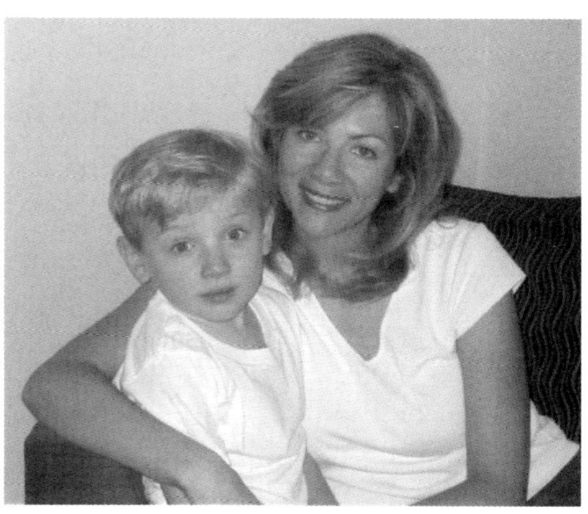

CONTACT:
elhautala@msn.com

Rohr was diagnosed at 3 years

Immediately after my son Rohr was born, the doctor placed him on my chest; we gazed into each other's eyes. I was astonished at the perfection of his body, the soulful wisdom in his newborn expression. I remember thinking, "this is the most significant moment of my life". I thanked God for giving me this blessing, this profound experience of joy; I thanked Him for sending me this tiny person who would change my life forever. Since then, there have been other significant moments in my life. Watching Rohr crawl, then take his first step; watching him smoosh his finger into the blue frosting on this first birthday cake. But none of those moments were as life altering as hearing the words "he's autistic" while my husband and I sat numbly in our chairs at Children's Hospital. There was no way to soften the blow of the doctor's diagnosis; there was no God to comfort me as I watched my hopes and dreams for my child's life unravel in an instant.

Oh sure, I'd known something was different about Rohr, almost from the beginning. When we brought him home from the hospital, his screaming would begin mid-afternoon and not cease until just before dawn. The times I was able to get him to look at me were few and far between. The new moms support group I joined was a burden to attend; every time I laid Rohr down on the floor with the other babies, he would immediately start screaming until I picked him up. Even though I dreaded going to the group in the beginning, watching the other babies develop differently than Rohr over time was one of my greatest blessings; it spurred me on to have him neurologically evaluated.

Once we received Rohr's diagnosis, his therapy plan was set in motion. The amount of services and hours required for his treatment were staggering to a mom who had expected to be filling her three-year-old son's schedule with "mommy and me" swim classes and library story hours; my rage at the impact of autism on my family and myself was all-consuming. I finally agreed to talk to a counselor, who gently urged me to see how all my hours spent engaging Rohr in interaction and transporting him to and from therapies was actually a blessing to our family. "Think of how bonded your relationship with him will be", she said.

I realize now, that had Rohr been a typical child, I might not have invested as much time getting to know and love him and all his idiosyncrasies. Ironically, the idiosyncrasies themselves may be the biggest blessings of all; within them, I see Rohr's phenomenal mind showing me beauty in a world I never knew existed. A world in which numbers dance together as beautifully as the patterns in an intricately hand-knitted sweater. A world in which loving, generous people such as therapists, program managers, and teachers show my son everyday that it's okay, even wonderful, to be different. It's true, my hopes and dreams for Rohr are different now than those I held for him as I gazed into his newborn eyes; but I wouldn't give up anything I've experienced with him in favor of a more "normal" life; there's been too many blessings along the way.

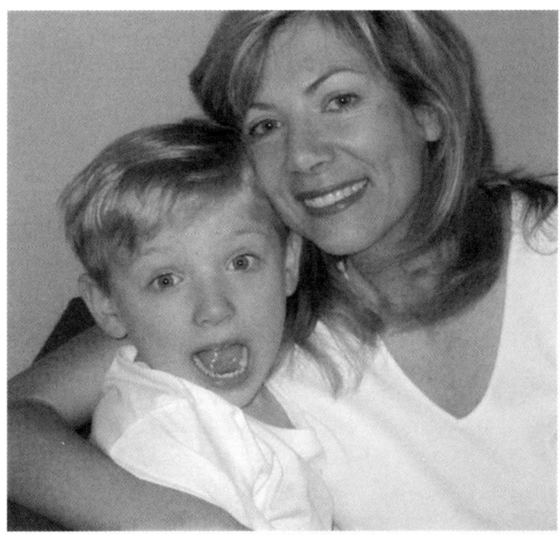

"I wouldn't give up anything I've experienced with him in favor of a more 'normal' life; there's been too many blessings along the way."

Maria & Drake

New Jersey

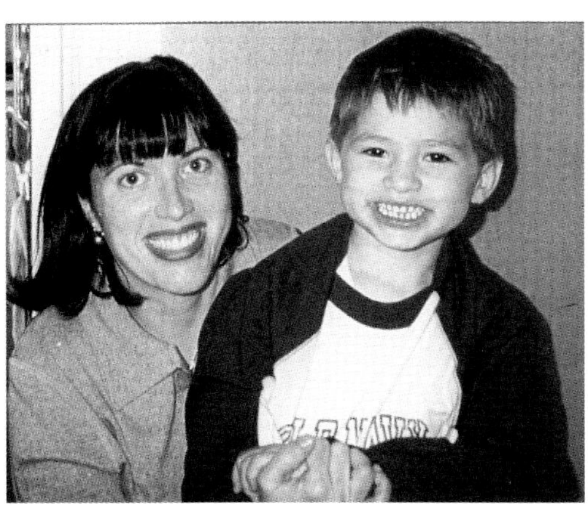

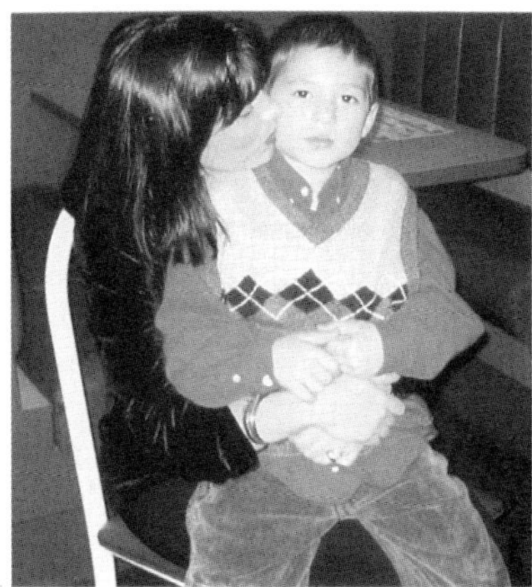

Drake, Thanksgiving 2004

CONTACT:
ionikos@peoplepc.com

Drake was diagnosed at 18 months

BIGGEST CHALLENGE(S)

Autism. The very word sends such varying emotions coursing through my body that it makes my mind reel at times. Just thinking back to Drake's diagnosis can bring me to my knees and remind me of days of blissful ignorance before this never-ending battle began. Long gone are the days when I didn't have to worry about every movement my son made; what could it mean? Never again are the days when I didn't have to worry about how his day was going to be; would he have a good therapy session?

Those carefree and worry-free days are forever lost. In their place are days filled with challenges, searching and pondering over what I should or could do to make my child better. It would probably be the moment that I began to give my son poison in his body (first, Rhogam injection) that would send him on this never-ending quest for recovery. If only I could alter these few blocks of time. If only there had been someone to warn me. Even so, would I have listened? Or would I have been just like those who look at me now as I warn them of the dangers of vaccinations, toxins and other things that can harm their baby. I can see it in their eyes; the look of pity and disbelief; "She's just crazy. She really thinks that there is a cure for her child." Even family members think that I have taken on a hopeless battle; a single knight with no army or support. Alone, fighting to bring back a body that could have been perfect; what God had really and truly created, rather than what man and chemicals have altered. It takes all my effort not to blame myself and wallow in self-pity. As educated and as well-read as I claim to be, how could I have let this happen? My only comfort is in knowing that this challenge must have been given to me to educate others and hope that within the hundreds that I "preach" to maybe one might listen.

My biggest challenge is truly seeing the possibility that there may be light at the end of this tunnel. Drake's accomplishments, though they may look tiny to others, are often huge for him. Easily they can bring tears of joy to my eyes. The first morning he woke up and called, "Mama," looking for me. The first time he tried to play a trick on me and I saw the twinkle in his eyes! The first time he finally began to write his name legibly. The first time I could show him a picture of a family member and he didn't say it was him! These are all things we take for granted as parents that we expect will automatically happen in a child's development. I take nothing for granted with Drake. Anything he accomplishes is a day of celebration, just as his failures can bring me down to the lowest possible point. It has been a long and hard battle. I still don't see an end in sight. I dare not look too far into the future. That would be much too much to bear. Those who know me, please have patience. I am the knight that will continue to fight until Drake's last symptom of autism is next to unrecognizable.

Greatest Blessings

I have to take a moment and thank a few people in Drake's life that have really made a difference. One is Drake's DAN doctor; Dr. Neubrander. He has been in our lives for three years. If it weren't for his never-ending research and dedication, Drake would not be where he is today. Drake's therapist, Rosemarie B. who never wavers no matter how "nutty" or torturous Drake can be. For myself, there is my friend, Laura, who just sits and listens to me rattle on about a connection between autism and vitamin/immune deficiency as an explanation to every behavior an autistic child might exhibit. My sister-in-law, Angie, who is more of a sister and the best friend I could ever have. Lastly, I'd like to thank my mom who listens to my crazy ranting on who is to blame for autism (mercury poisoning) and for the financial support she provides to help alleviate the burden on my family. And finally, to my husband who supports all my efforts to cure our son.

Words of Wisdom

For those just beginning this courageous battle, hold tight and never leave the fight. It will not be an easy campaign, yet you will have no choice but to forge ahead. Please take heart that there are many others just like you fighting the same battle and will see you at the end, victorious!

Favorite Resources:

1) *A Work in Progress* by Ron Leaf and John McEachin
2) *The Natural Medicine Guide to Autism* by Stephanie Marohn
3) *You're Going to Love This Kid!* by Paula Kluth
4) DAN (Defeat Autism Now) They have given all parents with autistic children a reason to hope that autism is curable.

Marie & Zack

Texas

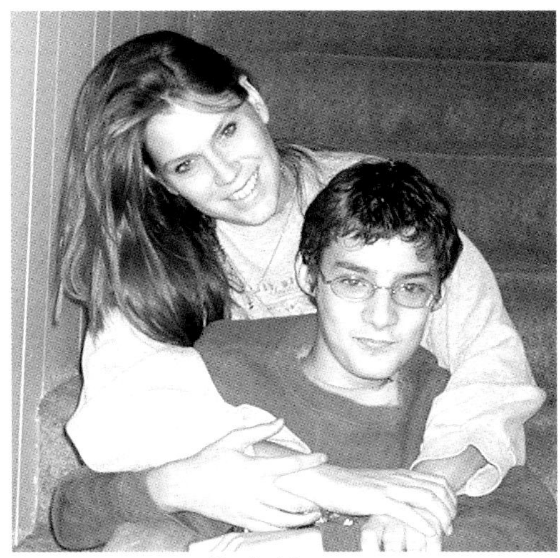

Zack 12 years

CONTACT:

whatruthinking2day@yahoo.com
mariemanning@msn.com

Zack was diagnosed at 3 years

BIGGEST CHALLENGE(S)

Zack used to walk down the street when he was one year old and tell me every make and model of every car he passed. However, he couldn't ask me for a drink of water or tell me he was hungry or cold, happy or sad. Rearranging expectations in those first years after we discovered he had autism was by far the hardest thing I have ever had to do. All of a sudden, the child who you thought was a genius is instead autistic. Expecting him to do the simplest thing like say "mom" or "I love you" had to be reexamined. I had to make a paradigm shift. Instead of placing expectations for him and his life, I had to expect myself to step up to the plate and learn how to accommodate and advocate for him. Those were hard and fast lessons in the beginning. All of a sudden I had to find resources and information on something I barely understood myself. The biggest struggle then, and still today, is knowing everything that is out there. It has been my experience that "you can't get it unless you know what it is and how to ask for it".

Greatest Blessings

At age twelve, there have been many funny stories and antics that had occurred over the years that have pulled us through. Zack's spirit and personality allow us to celebrate his differences, which often become the pillar of strength for us. I have fond memories of the first time Zack put his shoes on to get ready for school: one boot and one sandal. When I asked him about it, he said "Let's just pretend it's a match." Or, the first soccer game he played with other children who have disabilities when he walked off the field yelling, "That was the most fun I've ever had losing!" I think though, by far the greatest blessing to he and I is his sister. She is two years younger than him and his greatest advocate. She pushes him when he doesn't want to go further and supports him when he does. Recently, she flew down the stairs in a wave of excitement yelling, "Mom! Zack said he was going to tell on me because I flipped his hat off!" Her words were not that of a typical brother/sister rivalry; but those of exuberance because he didn't react negatively toward her when she tried to provoke him.

Words of Wisdom

The road families must take when they have a child with autism is not the same as "The Jones's". Each day brings with it unique challenges that cannot be compared to the daily life of families who do not understand what a picture exchange system is or why you are allowing your child to read a magazine at the zoo. Discern what is right for your family and go for it. There are always going to be those who will never understand what life is like living with a child who has autism. Always remember that you are your child's biggest advocate and with that information is the key. The more you can learn, the more you can fight for the needs of your child. Be proactive in your pursuit to education, community services and access. However, be wary of fads and misinformation. Understand how the Americans with Disabilities Act and the Individuals with Disabilities Education Act (IDEA) can serve your child. Also, understand how the local school system works. Most important, pick your battles wisely. There is no need to fight over the little things when the bigger picture is at stake. Finally, ensure that other family members are not left out while the focus is on one. The more involved the family becomes in the pursuit of life the closer the family will become.

Favorite Resources:

1) www.nichy.org (nationwide)
2) www.wrightslaw.com (nationwide)
3) www.arc.org (nationwide)
4) *Thinking in Pictures* by Temple Grandin
5) *A Work in Progress* by Leaf and McEachin

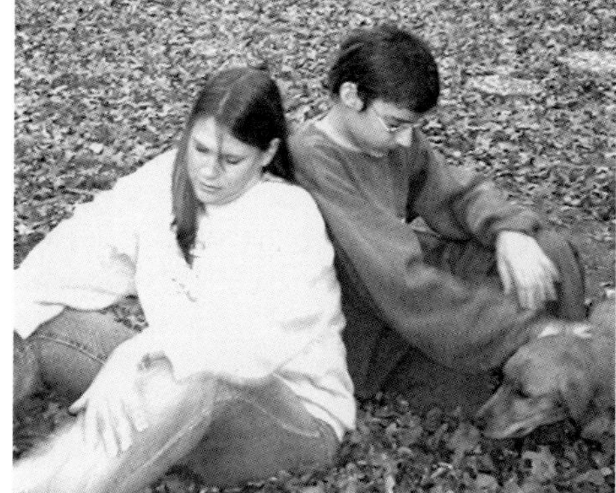

Melody & Mark

Kansas

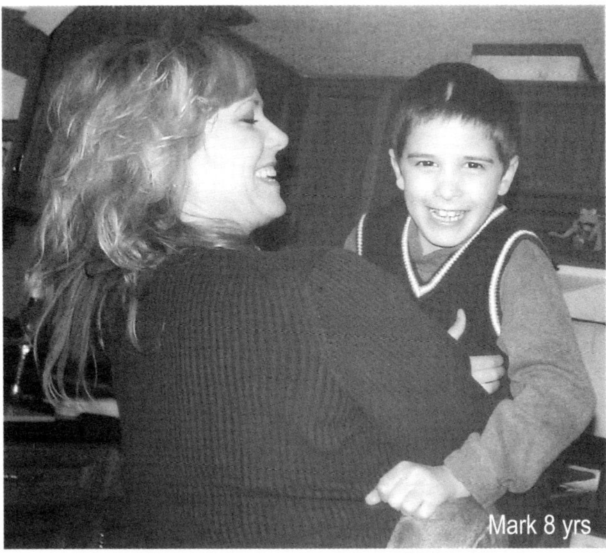
Mark 8 yrs

CONTACT:
MetsinKs@aol.com

Mark was diagnosed at 2½ years

BIGGEST CHALLENGE(S)

I would first like to say that as a parent of a child with special needs there are so many challenges on a daily basis to face. It's being able to still laugh and love life that make the challenges less stressful and almost a neccssity to keep trudging the water that is still so full of ripples in this particular special need.

I think the biggest challenge at first was getting used to all the providers and therapists invading my home and parenting. After time you realize some of these people have a wonderful gift and are helping you and your family. It's almost comforting to have someone to share things with and a common ground, which is your child's best interest being met.

Other challenges along the way you may encounter may be eating habits, sleeping habits, time for therapy, getting enough therapy or overloading your child with too much therapy, adequate therapists and all the appointments with doctors and school officials.

My future challenge, which brings me to tears, is what will be available for my son when he is older. Perhaps a resident home or placement. A decision I'm not looking forward to making. This is where having such wonderful people in my life to lean on is almost a necessity.

I look at it like this; despite his diagnosis I find whatever help is out there for him. And if that diagnosis gets him more help, great. He lives full-time with his sister and three step-siblings and step-dad and myself, his mom. He is still non-verbal despite years of speech therapy and early intervention at the house and through school. He may never be potty trained or ride a bike without training wheels. He has certain foods he will not touch. But I will never give up the fight of trying and working with him.

Greatest Blessings

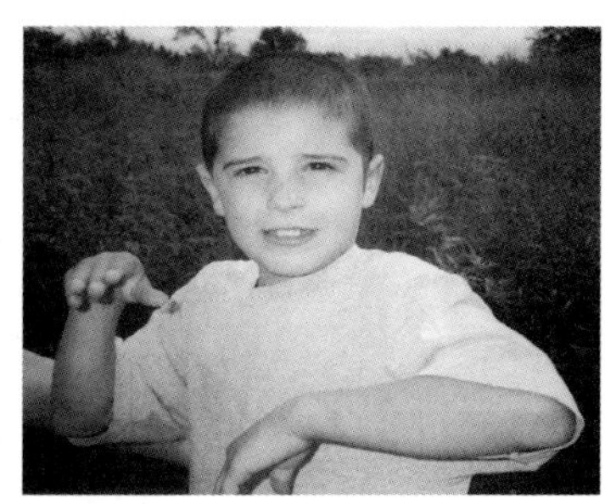

My blessings in life are still on-going. Just being Markie's Mom brightens up my day. What he has managed to teach me is priceless and couldn't have been done by anyone else. Having three step-children and my daughter who don't treat him too much differently, for that Markie is blessed as well.

I'm blessed to have family in both Kansas and Pennsylvania that are so supportive in my life and Mark's. My husband Matt, Markie's step-dad, is the rock and stability that this kind of parenting needs. It truly takes a special heart to love unconditionally a child that is not yours and on top of that has special needs. For all these wonderful things I am blessed. Some days you need to look hard for blessings and other days they just fall in your lap. It depends on how you choose to see the day at hand.

Words of Wisdom

If I could offer words of wisdom it would be to never stop learning from your child, only then can you give proper therapies and be his biggest advocate. Surround yourself with positive, loving family and people. Never close your doors no matter how painful the occasion may be. Never lose hope and reality. I like to say I'm 50% hope and 50% reality; I have to be for Mark. Choose to be happy and enjoy the time God has given you with your child. And some days it is a hard choice; that is where wonderful friends and family help out.

> "Some days you need to look hard for blessings and other days they just fall in your lap."

Favorite Resources:

1) *The Autistic Spectrum Parents Daily Helper* by Philip Abrams and Leslie Henriques
2) *Let Me Hear Your Voice* by Katherine Maurice (she also has a workbook available)
3) *The Ride Together* by Paul and Judy Karasik
4) *Son Rise the Miracles Continues* by Barry Kaufman
5) Anything to do with Wright's law
6) *Children with Autism/A Parents Guide* edited by Michael D. Powers Psy.D

Michelle & Brandon

Texas

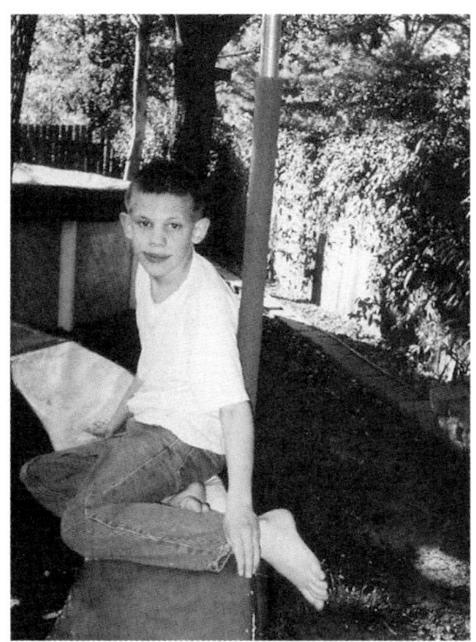

Brandon was diagnosed at 18 months

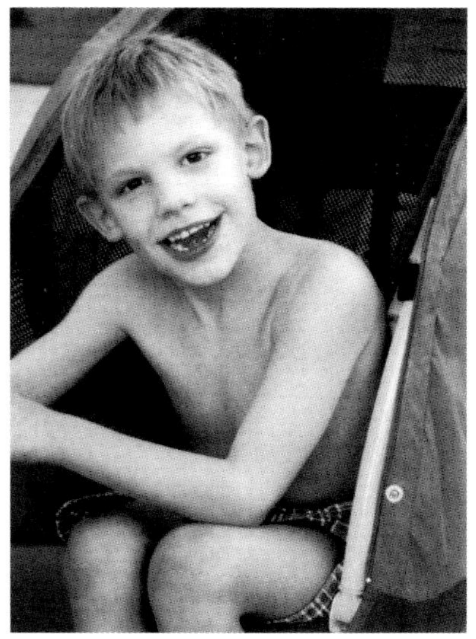

Contact:
MichelleMGuppy@yahoo.com
www.TexasAutismAdvocacy.org

Just Breathe

Most people can remember the day President Kennedy was shot. They know when it was, where they were, what they were doing. It was a moment forever impressed on their memory.

Parents of special needs children have memories like that — whether it was the moment in the pediatrician's office when they first heard the news — or sometime later when the reality hit. Either way, it is a moment that forever changes them. I remember the day that the reality of my son's diagnosis hit me – for me, it wasn't the day he was diagnosed with the disorder. At that time, in the pediatrician's office, it wasn't a shock. I had felt that Mother's instinct that there were things not right, that my child was a bit delayed and had some odd behaviors. But when the pediatrician gave the condition and concerns a name I felt more relief than shock. "Autism", he said. I didn't know what Autism was — I didn't know anyone with it — but I was relieved. Because now I could go buy a book, do what it said, and my son would be healed. I thought all would be well.

I found out all too soon that this was a bit more complicated than I thought, but still, I was hopeful. I learned all I could on my own and I enrolled my child in every therapy and special school that was recommended. Looking back, I realize that during those first few months after my son's diagnosis reality had not set in. I don't even think I was shocked. I was too ignorant of the disorder. I just knew that there was a "name" for the disorder my son had and so if I just tried hard enough I could "cure" it. Then I met Mitchell…and I saw reality.

A playgroup was recommended by my son's teacher. She said her son with autism attended that program and was really doing well there. Her son Mitchell was 13, and my son was 3 at the time. I enrolled my son, and was hopeful. I looked forward to the program and to meeting Mitchell.

The day came to take my little boy to the playgroup and I walked in all excited for my child and anxious to meet Mitchell. I got my child settled in his age group, and asked where I could find Mitchell. An attendant pointed to a room with a video playing – and there was Mitchell. A tall, handsome 13-year-old boy, flying an imaginary airplane and repeating the same phrase over and over. I walked up to him and said hello, thinking he hadn't noticed me. He never looked at me, he just kept flying his imaginary airplane and repeating the same phrase over and over. Reality hit. It hit really hard.

I ran to my car in tears and just sat there in the parking lot and cried and cried and cried. I screamed. I begged God. I bargained with God. And I got angry with God. Then I cried until my chest felt so tight that I couldn't breathe. The reality of my son's diagnosis sunk in that day in the car. It was the day my dreams for my son were shot. And it was a day I would never forget.

I was in the car in the parking lot for over an hour, and when I could cry no more, I thought, "If I just stop breathing, this will all go away. If I don't take that next breath, I won't have to face this reality. I can make this moment of horror stop." Obviously if you stop breathing, you stop living. But I didn't want to die. I just wanted how I felt to die, to stop, to not go on. I didn't want to face the reality that my son, might grow up to be like her son. In the quiet of that moment it felt as if God was saying, "Michelle, if you will just breathe….if you just take that next breath, you can go on. Each breath you take will help you through this…" And so I listened to that voice. I didn't want to; I fought it, even held my breath for a moment longer. But I listened and breathed one painful breath after another. And have been doing so everyday since then…

My son is now 9-years-old, still non-verbal, and still autistic. I have been blessed abundantly by him in so many countless ways. He has been a blessing to the countless lives that he has touched. He has come so far and overcome so many obstacles! There were of course, times when it was hard — when I wanted to just stop breathing to make it all go away. What kept, and will keep, me going is remembering that voice from God in the car so long ago…. "Just Breathe…" And I do.

The Butterfly

The picture in my mind that represents the biggest challenge and greatest blessing of having autism in my life is that of a butterfly. For me, the butterfly represents the transformation of my life from before autism to my life after autism. Those first few years after Brandon was diagnosed with autism were hard to say the least. My hopes and dreams for my son as a "typical" child were shattered. I felt like a "crippled caterpillar" who wanted nothing more than to hide in a cocoon and not ever come out. Obviously that wasn't an option.

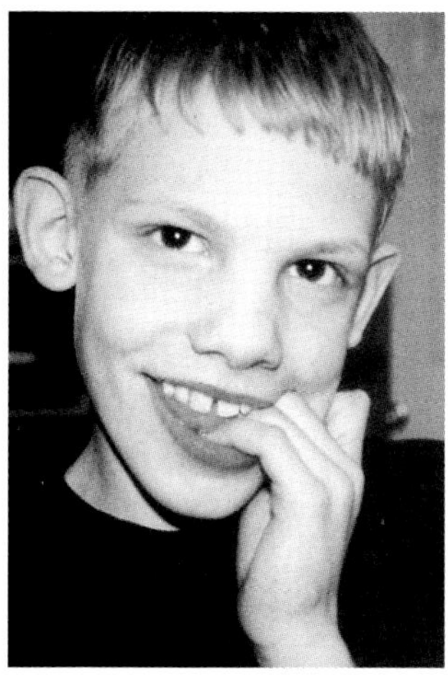

During many tearful nights in prayer, and thanks to God's grace and mercy, my attitude was transformed from despair to hope. I believe it is Sally Meyer's tagline that reads, "Autism is not the end of the world, it's the beginning of a new one, just open your eyes, and see." And so I did.

Slowly, I began to emerge from that cocoon of devastation, despair, anger, self-pity, and all the other emotions that were swirling in my head. Slowly my eyes were opened to the beauty of my child and in the many blessings of this new life. I found new friends in my community and hundreds of internet friends that I have never met, but only know by their e-mail address. My transformation was in realizing for the first time what matters most in life and what unconditional love is. In letting go and letting God. My husband's transformation was in learning how to accept that which he could not fix or change. He learned the humility of being on his knees crying to God for help. My typical son Matthew's transformation was that he has become a more mature, compassionate, unselfish, big brother. His prayers at night suddenly went from, "God bless my Mom and Dad and please let me have a new bicycle" to ; "God please help someone unlock autism so my brother can talk and all the children with autism can be cured." He asks me if I have been saving money for when they do unlock autism, so we can afford the cure.

Perhaps the most profound transformation has been in those touched by Brandon. That has been incredible to witness. So many lives this silent, autistic, child of mine has touched! Their lives would not have been transformed had it not been for Brandon and his life with autism. Acceptance is liberation, not defeat.

The caterpillar was designed by the creator to one day become a butterfly. To accept that there is purpose in my child having autism is to know true peace. I don't have to agree with it or like it, but I must accept it. Psalm 139 says, "All the days ordained for me were written in your book before one of them came to be..." Whether by vaccination, genetics, poisons in the environment, whatever; God knew my child would be the way he is. I am not defeated by accepting that. I am instead liberated. Free to start from that point forward in making my child's life be the best it can possibly be. Free to help other parents with what I have learned. Free to make my voice heard in support of research, legislation, and services for my child. Free to know that it's not up to me whether one day he flies or not, but to simply encourage him, help him, and give him every opportunity to try. Free to know that whether my child is cured or not, I did my very best for him. It's a hard journey, but we have a choice.

Even the butterfly must struggle to get out of it's cocoon, and once out, there are predators and windshields out there to avoid! So make no mistake, our journey has not been easy, nor will it probably ever be easy. As with any situation in life, there are good days and there are bad days. But we have a choice... We can choose to focus on the ugliness of autism and the limitations and challenges it brings, which can be crippling; or we can choose to focus on the beauty and blessings of our child and what he can do. I choose beauty (and a good sense of humor about it all!).

God's Beautiful Butterfly

by Michelle M. Guppy

I am a child who has Autism,
who may not do things exactly like you.
But that does not mean I am useless,
I have feelings and emotions, just like you.

I can hear the things you are saying,
even though with words I cannot yet speak.
I may not be able to play sports like you,
but that does not mean I am weak.

I know there are many things about me,
that you simply do not understand.
But please don't shy away from me,
talk to me and perhaps offer to shake my hand.

I may have a mind that works differently,
pages in a book – I may flap instead of turn;
But that does not mean you can't teach me,
you might be surprised at just what I can learn.

If you think when I don't cooperate, I'm misbehaving,
and conclude that I'm not disciplined enough;
please take a moment to consider,
that the road I am traveling can be tough.

When you stare at me, point, or start to whisper,
It makes me sad, and I so want to cry ---
Why do you view me as some crippled caterpillar?
Why can't you see that I'm God's beautiful butterfly?

Monica & Alex

New York

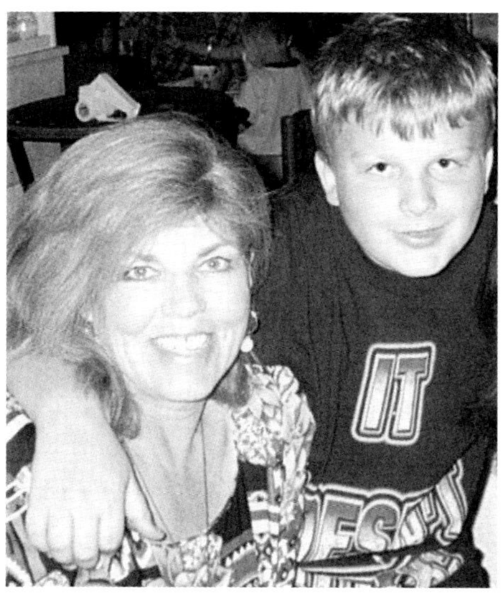

Alex was diagnosed at 4 years

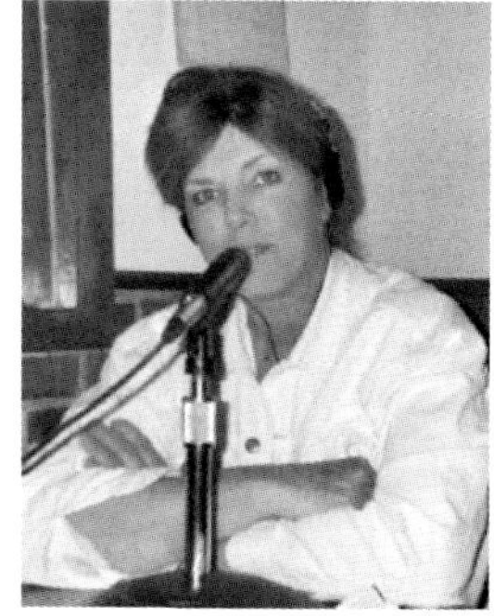

CONTACT:
monica@poweradvocates.org and
monica@disabilitynewsradio.com
www.disabilitynewsradio.com

BIGGEST CHALLENGE(S)

There were several "big" challenges when my son Alexander was first identified as a child with a learning disability. He was only four years old then. While Alex didn't appear to look disabled, he exhibited different behaviors than his older twin brother and sister had when they were the same age. Alex interacted well with adults, and especially one-on-one, but displayed concerns when he was with other children and peers in group settings at the daycare he was attending. He reacted to sounds more drastically (i.e., fire alarms, balloons popping, and fireworks) than most children. He was clearly sensitive to clothing (shirts, tags, collars, socks and certain textures) along with certain foods too. Once it was apparent that Alex's social skills, along with the sensory issues, were affecting him; I began reading, researching books and the internet, and joining various groups online to help identify my son's challenges.

My problem was in accepting my baby, my youngest, had anything "wrong" with him. He looked so perfect with his bright blue eyes and blond hair! The camera loved Alex and Alex loved the camera! Alex had modeled at 12 months of age and appeared on several toy boxes.

Another huge challenge was to trust the professionals and administrators that I had met with who seemed to "care" about my son, like I did. As a parent, I looked up to these people as experts in their respective fields (psychologists, nurses, teachers, medical doctors, and school staff). While I had hoped that the professionals that were part of my son's assessments and ultimately his diagnosis would be able to answer my questions, and ultimately solve my son's problems, little did I realize that I, and my faith in God, were going to be a bigger part of the help and answers to help my son Alex.

Another big challenge for me, and many parents who become part of the Special Education system, is not knowing what your rights are for your child under Federal (IDEA) and State laws. Thankfully, I was able to find an experienced and caring parent advocate named Sheila who held my hand and answered my ongoing questions about the Special Education laws and how these applied specifically in my son's life, his IEP, and future.

Greatest Blessings

As a single mom at 40 years young, having Alex has taught me to trust God more in life, especially in adversity. Alex has shown me a new world, a better world which people (children and adults) with disabilities live. I have found Alex to be kinder, more loving, gentle, and always forgiving – traits that I am sure God would want us to exhibit. Often times, we spend our lives trying to achieve these, or some of these, qualities. Alexander has had these qualities all along!

Words of Wisdom

Follow your own instincts. Read, research, listen, pray, accept, love, forgive, trust God, pray, dream, believe and use your experiences to help make a difference in other people's lives!

My favorite scripture from the Bible:

"For I know the plans I have for you, declares the Lord, plans for welfare and not for calamity, to give you a future and a hope." Jeremiah 29:11

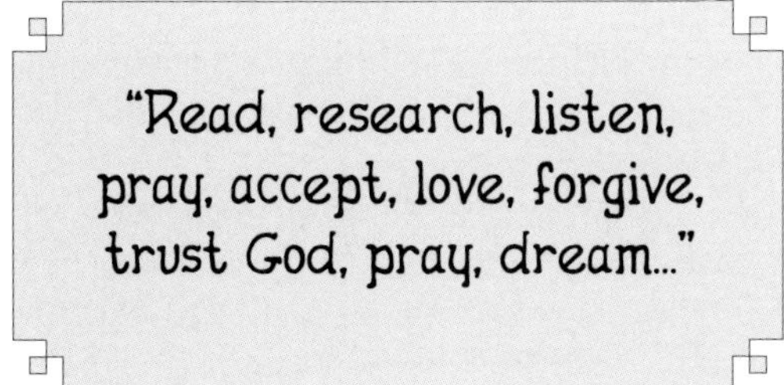

Monique & Kenny

Georgia

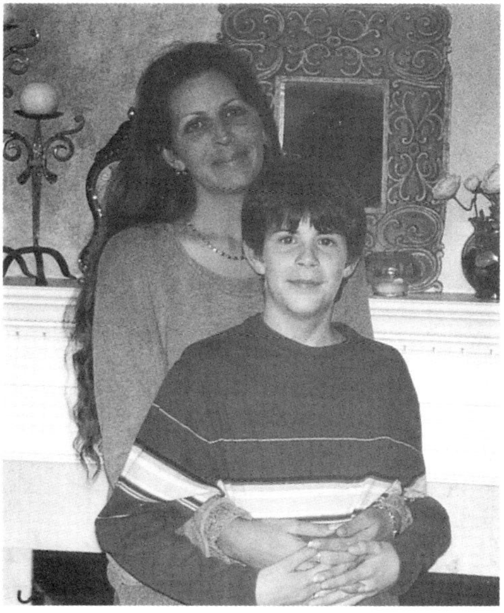

Kenny was diagnosed Asperger's at 10 years

Biggest Challenge(s)

I would have to say that our biggest first challenge was a correct diagnosis. From age 5 on, everyone had their own opinion of what was going on, and of course the schools just want to medicate. Our current challenge is still school, and everyone's ten-cent opinion on how to "fix" things. It is amazing how people think they can see someone for 5 minutes and rule out so many things that Mommy could not possibly have heard before.

Our personal challenges are the more worrisome ones. Trying to see things Kenny's way is very hard, trying to make sense of his social skills is heartbreaking. Hoping for the future is almost exhausting. Repeating myself, and reminding myself of his level of understanding is frustrating. People ignoring him is the all-time worst. I fear for him being taken advantage of. The teen years ahead scare me to death. I want him to feel comfortable in his own skin, to have self-esteem. I want him to see himself like I see him — wonderful.

Greatest Blessings

My greatest blessing is having my children and a wonderful husband to keep me together. It is a blessing to have the ability to help yourself help your child. I am blessed by my beautiful daughter, who has the ability to speak her mind and protect. I love the moments of any kind of accomplishment that Kenny makes and is proud of. I love to see him smile. He is my first, and he is a good boy, just misunderstood. The greatest blessing is to one day have acceptance from anyone he comes in contact with, and the world not be afraid of "special". My friends, also in the spectrum, Irene and Jeannie are treasures and irreplaceable. I am blessed for a supportive family.

Words of Wisdom

My words of wisdom are:

- Run from the word "denial", it only wastes time.
- These children need our voices, and we need help.
- I have learned more from other parents than anyone else.
- Empower yourself with knowledge.
- Don't back down with the schools……
- Thank God for support groups and great friends!

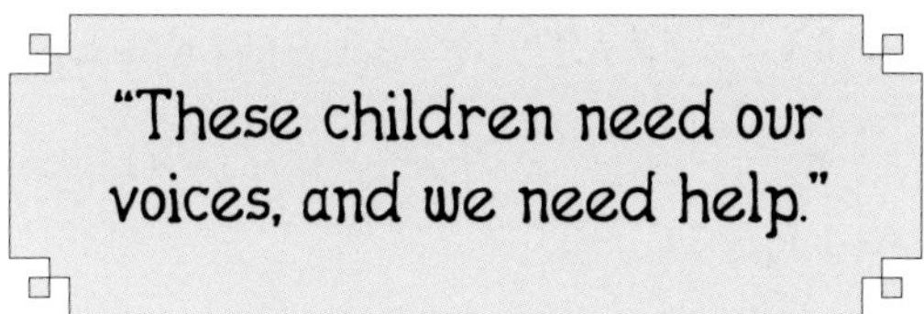

Favorite Resources:

1) www.cureautismnow.org (please donate ☺)
2) kidesteem@aol.com This is for Lee and Marianne Chasen, the "masters of social skills groups", on Long Island, NY, also author of my favorite book, *The Sacred Weave of Mothering*, a heartfelt thank you for all of my power, and the continuing long distance support!
3) http://groups.yahoo.com/group/AspergerAutism_Teens Support for Aspie's
4) http://pub6.bravenet.com/forum/445720254/show/297577 Support for siblings
5) http://www.udel.edu/bkirby/asperger/grandparents.html For Grandparents!
6) http://www.autismshop.com Great things!
7) http://www.iep4u.com Great advice for IEPs

Nicole & James

Wisconsin

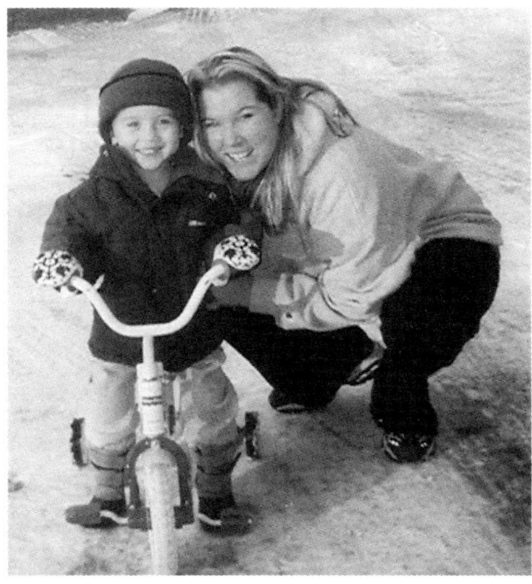

Contact:
connorn@nlg.com

James was diagnosed at 3 years

Biggest Challenge(s)

Trying to find ways to comfort my non-verbal child when I cannot always figure out what's wrong.

Greatest Blessings

Every smile, every laugh, every time we get eye contact, and sometimes, only sometimes if you look close enough there is a sparkle in their eye no matter how small, it's there.

Words of Wisdom

One day at a time, understanding some days will be one hour at a time. Focus on today not always tomorrow or the 'what ifs'. Our son James wakes up with a smile and goes to bed with one, so we must be doing something right.

Imagine

by Nicole Lannyk

Imagine
No "I love yous"
No family picnics, parades, or weddings,
No friends or playmates,
No common sense.

Imagine
A 4-year-old that doesn't understand what
will happen if he runs in front of a car
or jumps into a pool.
Imagine a home looking like Ft. Knox
just to keep your child safe.

Imagine
Being told your child has a neurological brain disorder
and maybe will never be able to speak, function in society,
live alone, marry or have children, your heart sinks.

Imagine
After waking your child in the morning, if you don't do
everything in the same order as the day before, at the
precise moment it's enough to ruin their entire day.

Imagine
Watching your child on the first day of school
stepping into the handicapped bus.

Imagine
Having your home invaded with teachers, therapists,
State reps, child psychologists for 35hrs per week of intense
1-on-1 therapy in hopes of a better life someday.

Imagine
Watching the agony on your child's face giving you the
"Mommy why are you letting them do this to me" look while
doing numerous EEG's, blood work, x-rays, and testing to
figure out how to help them feel better.

Imagine
Just how many "your kids a brat" stares you get in public
simply because your child cannot handle social situations
including a simple trip to the grocery store.
Imagine
What autistic children, parents and families go through
on a daily basis.

Nicole & Khalid

Oregon

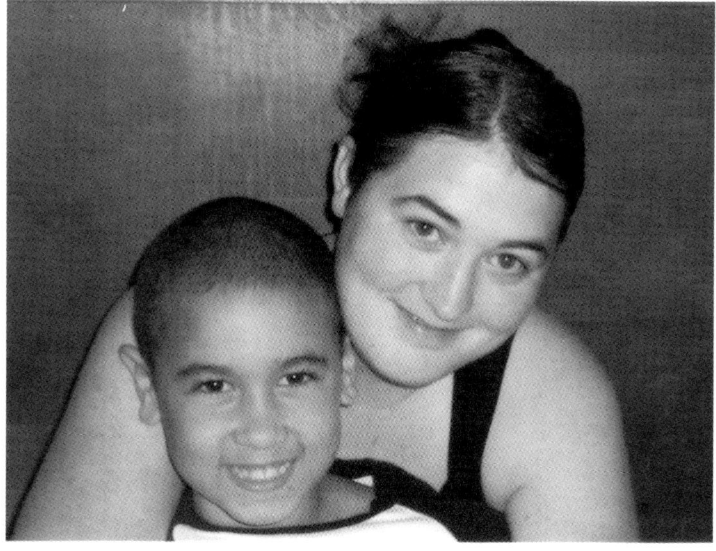

Khalid was diagnosed Asperger's at 7 years

Biggest Challenge(s)

My son was diagnosed with Asperger's Syndrome at age seven and the biggest challenge I face is a lack of understanding, or the desire to understand. People are so quick to judge a child that is different, a child that has social difficulties that they cannot imagine.

As my son gets older, the social gap that didn't seem to matter much in kindergarten has now widened and I am very aware of how difficult life can be. A friend that once came over every chance he got is now socially more mature and has moved on; another friend lost.

Some family members who once seemed supportive now show their annoyance; the tolerance and solace once available can no longer be assumed. Summer camps and classes cannot handle the difficulty and rigidity that often escalate to a rage — doors of opportunity closed to a boy who loves to learn.

I know that no matter how wonderful and talented and amazing my son is, there are so many people that cannot or will not see this. At times I want to scream out loud! Yes, my son is different, but that does not make him any less extraordinary.

GREATEST BLESSINGS

One of the greatest blessings in my life is my son's love. I have learned new meanings of the word love by accepting Khalid as he is and opening my heart...

Love is...
the warmth of his tears streaming down my cheek
as he hugs me tight and tells me why his heart hurts.

Love is...
the pounding of his feet
as he races towards me when I pick him up from school.

Love is...
the curiosity his mind reveals
in the hundreds of questions he asks each day.

Love is...
the sound of his laughter filling the air,
encouraging me to laugh aloud with him.

Love is...
the tug of his fingers pulling me in the direction of his latest discovery.

Love is...
the twinkle of his eyes as he wakes me up on a Saturday morning.

Love is...
everything he is, and everything he means to me.

From the tip of his head, to the bottom of his toes, my son is perfect to me.

WORDS OF WISDOM

I have some simple words of advice:

Love your child and embrace your life. Autism is not the end of the world, but it is a new world. Accepting a journey you didn't intend to take requires courage and perseverance. Along the way you will encounter fear of the unknown, anger at bullies and mean kids, exasperation at jumping through hoops to get the help and services needed at school, and the pain of rejection, both of your child and yourself. Do not give up! Your child needs you, and up the road there also awaits the excitement of a new friend you made, joy from seeing the firsts: first basketball shot made, first crush, first dance; beauty in watching your child do what they do best (because we all have special talents!), and relief in discovering you are not alone. Dreams don't have to end; sometimes they just change.

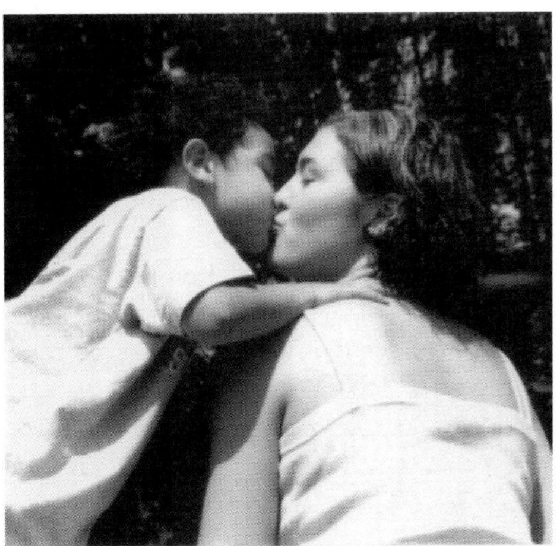

Pam & Evan

Kansas

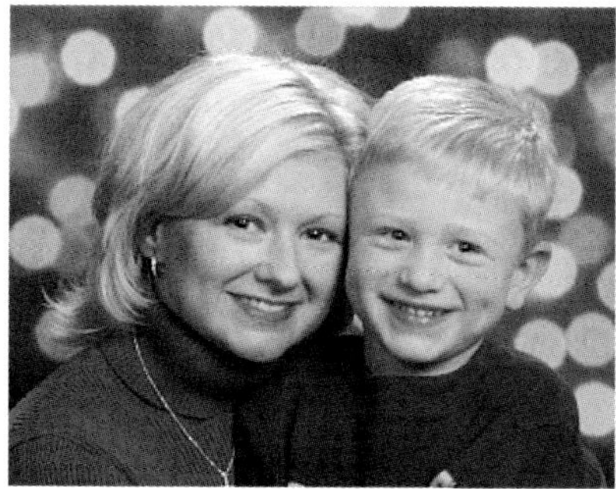

CONTACT:
Pamela.wells@labone.com

Evan was diagnosed at 3½ years

BIGGEST CHALLENGE(S)

I would have to say there are a variety of challenges in raising a child with autism...some bigger than others. One of them would be trying to balance your life so that it is healthy for everyone involved. It is so easy to get so preoccupied with trying to find every single thing that you possibly can to help your child, that you lose sight of stopping to just let him be a child. I have found that it is so important to take time to just be. What I mean by that is taking time to really enjoy every moment you have with him/her. If you let yourself become obsessed with researching every little thing you can, then you might just miss some special moments.

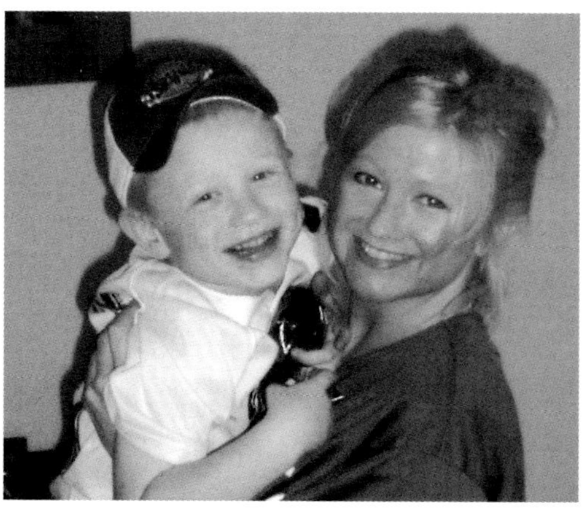

Greatest Blessings

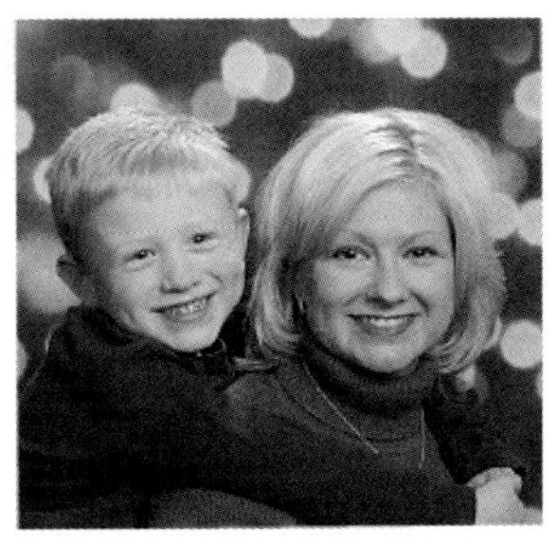

I don't even know where to begin with this... My son, Evan and I have been truly blessed by so many people. To start, I would have to say that one of Evan's "Angels" would be his Grandma Kathy and Grandpa Gary. They have been by both our sides through thick and thin and have always seen Evan's full potential – before he ever reaches it. I have to thank a few more "Angels" in Evan's life that have made a tremendous difference not only in his life, but in mine as well. They will never know how much I appreciate all of their dedication with the many challenges that Evan has overcome. So, thank you to Aida (preschool teacher), Joan D. (OT/PT therapist), and Alison (speech language pathologist). It is so important to find special people like the ones Evan and I have worked with to make a true difference in your child.

I think that Evan himself is one of my greatest blessings. I would not change a thing about him even if I could. He has the most beautiful outlook that I have ever seen in any child, especially a child with challenges. He will put a smile on your face as soon as he walks into the room. He is my Angel.

Words of Wisdom

My only words of wisdom would be to stay positive and don't take no for an answer. Do everything within your power to utilize every source you can that will help your child today and tomorrow. There will be days when you feel like giving up...and as soon as you start to feel that way, your child will do yet another thing that truly amazes you and you have the motivation to go on forever. Do your best and know that your child is capable of so much more than you can imagine. Last, but not least, love your child. I am thankful that I have been given the opportunity to share my thoughts with you.

"If you let yourself become obsessed with researching every little thing you can, then you might just miss some special moments."

Phyllis & Anthony

Washington

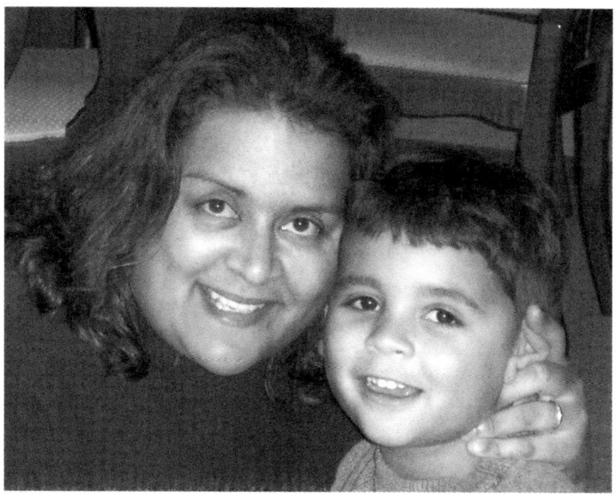

CONTACT:
Dzerman2@yahoo.com

Anthony was diagnosed at 26 months

BIGGEST CHALLENGE(S)

Autism for me has been like a dark shadow that crept in late one night and stole not only my son, but my dreams. Dreams of how we would play, share in long bike rides, travel and explore the world. Dreams of him growing into a young man who was popular and athletic. Dreams of him getting married and me becoming a grandmother. Dreams for the best in life. Anthony's diagnosis of autism not only stole my child, it also stole my dreams. Without dreams there is only an unknown darkness lurking on the horizon — ready to snatch the joys of every day, minute, hour and second. The present becomes not a gift to unwrap but a moment to endure another day of lost dreams. The greatest challenge for me is to keep moving forward and redefining my dream according to the person Anthony is slowly revealing himself to be. The boy, the dreams and purpose he is designed to fulfill is now bittersweet. I have come to accept this death of my dreams. Yet, like death of any type there are stages of grief that come and go like the tide according to life events. The greatest challenge in letting go of my dreams and illusions is not mourning the loss, but celebrating in the revelations of today.

Greatest Blessings

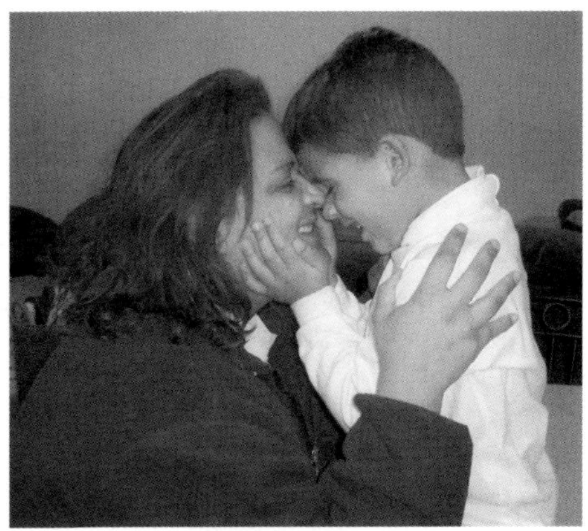

Anthony 5 years old

I feel one of the greatest gifts in life is being able to find the light in the valley of the darkness. Autism for many of us is just that…a long valley filled with darkness. The journey through the diagnosis, the loss of dreams, the redefining of life as I know it, certainly are the moments of darkness. I have grown immensely from the trials of autism in my life. The greatest blessing of my journey is the new found ability to celebrate! Celebration not only comes in the form of good grades or winning touchdowns, but in trying a new food or babbling a new string of sounds. As the twinkle in my son's eye shows life and growth, I celebrate. After two years I finally heard my son say "Momma", I celebrate. When he started to protest with the word "No", I celebrate. When he spoke the cherished words "I love you", I celebrate. When his eyes light up with a mischievous glimmer and he teases me or his sister, I celebrate. Autism has caused a reshuffling of my priorities and the way I look at life. With the diagnosis came the great gift to celebrate like few do by rejoicing in the little things in life. Even when life seems difficult and I cannot see through the darkness, my child will come to me and wrap his arms around my neck, I know that I can celebrate all over again.

Words of Wisdom

My song in life has been "Don't waste your pain". Through these hard earned words of wisdom I have been able to move forward, starting support groups, sharing information and most importantly, remembering what it felt like the first time I heard the word autism used to describe Anthony. I have dedicated my life to the sharing and support of families who are just starting this journey. I have turned my pain into something positive that I can give back to those who are hurting. I have been strengthened by giving. I have been comforted by comforting. I have been blessed by sharing my blessing.

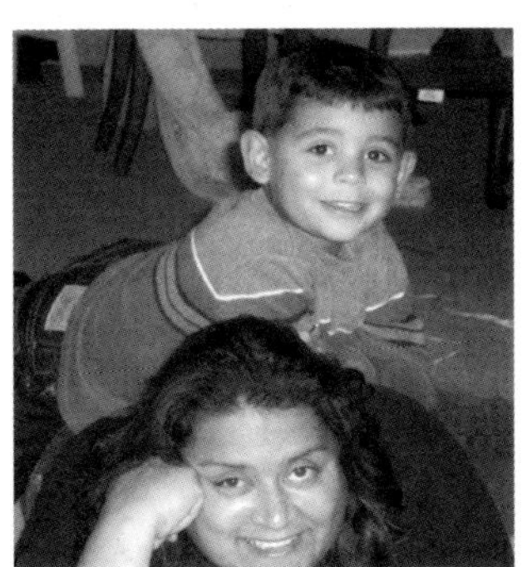

My word's of wisdom to share: **"Don't turn inward, turn outward. Don't waste your pain".**

Rachel & Tyler

Georgia

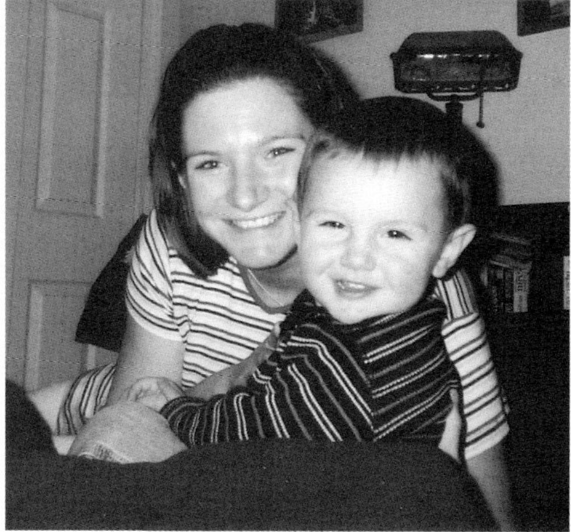

Tyler at 23 months

Contact:
tylerhaley01@alltel.net

Tyler was diagnosed at 3 years

Biggest Challenge(s)

I have had a few challenges but I think that the greatest challenge is trying not to worry too much. I can't count the nights I have sat beside my son's bed and cried because his future is so uncertain.

Greatest Blessings

The greatest blessing for me is the way that my family has been so supportive. From my mother wearing her autism awareness bracelet to my brother who changed his college major so that he could be a special education teacher.

Words of Wisdom

Don't fret over the things you can't change. Just give your child the patience and love that only a mother can. My brother told me when we found out that our son was autistic: "God chose you to be Tyler's mom because he knew you were the best one for the job." The same is true for every mother with an autistic child.

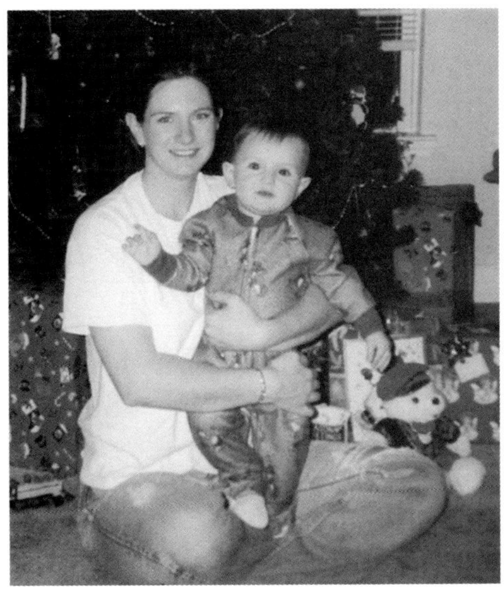

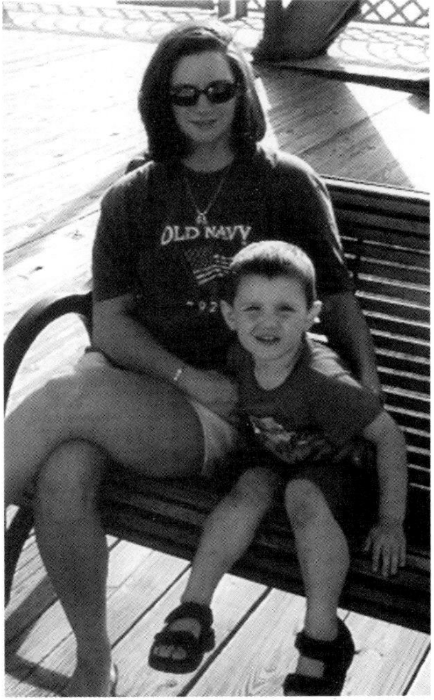

Tyler 3 years old

Favorite Resources:

Facing Autism by Lynn M. Hamilton

> "Life is not measured
> by the breaths
> we take,
> but by the moments
> that take
> our breath away."
>
> – Anonymous

Ruthie & Mandy

New Mexico

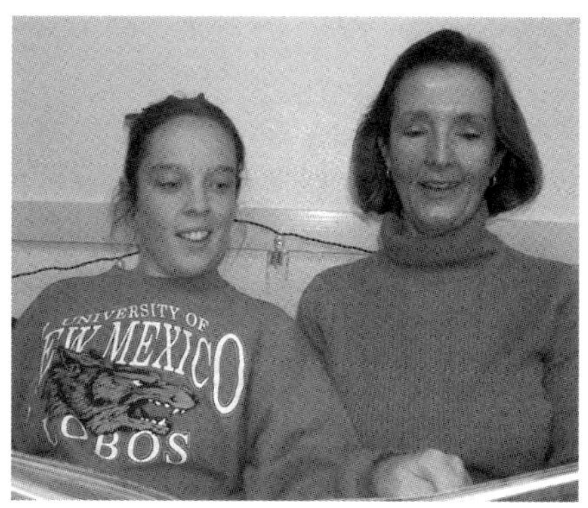

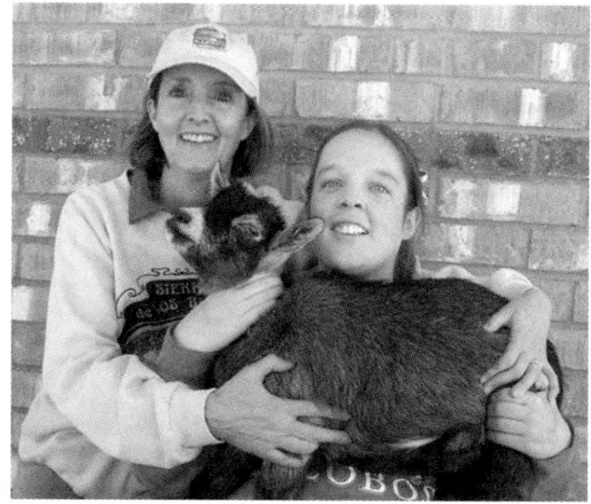

Mandy was diagnosed at 11 years

CONTACT:

drmrobb@worldnet.att.net

www.MandysFarm.org

BIGGEST CHALLENGE(S)

Our daughter was born in 1982, but was not diagnosed as a person with autism for another eleven years. I first knew that something was wrong when, after having a major vaccine reaction at 18 months of age, she began losing skills that she had previously acquired. Not knowing what was wrong was one of my biggest challenges as I tried to find appropriate therapy and to see to it that she was moving forward in her development. No one could tell me what was wrong or what I needed to do for her. With the stresses of Mandy's behavior, keeping our family together was difficult at best. Eventually, when she was four, I had to leave my career to care for her and my family. However, providing this care left me constantly tired from dealing with therapists, Mandy's behavior outbursts and trying to advance her development. This left me with no time for anything else—certainly not for me. Mandy also suffers from major grand mal seizures that, during her early years, were not controlled and left both of us exhausted and scared. Fortunately, we were eventually able to bring them under control with appropriate medication.

Greatest Blessings

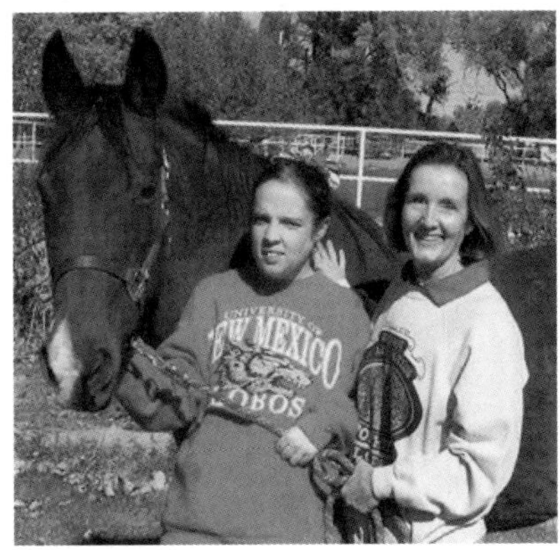

Mandy is probably the happiest person I know. She taught me to look at what is really important in life, which in turn made me a better person and parent. I learned to appreciate the little things that we often take for granted in each other and in the world. I came to realize that even small triumphs were something to be celebrated. I have also been blessed by the wonderful people we never would have met if Mandy had not had autism. They have made our lives fuller and they remain friends to her and to me to this day.

Words of Wisdom

Trust your gut. You are your child's parent and you know him or her better than anyone else. You are the best advocate for your child, so don't let others push you into making a decision for your child that you know is not the right thing. If you feel you are doing the right thing, trust yourself and go with it. Make time for yourself no matter how you have to do it. Don't lose yourself completely in taking care of those around you. If you overextend yourself, then you won't be of use to anyone much less your child with autism who desperately needs you. While these children are intense, don't let them become your entire world. Also don't forget to plan for the future. Our children will grow up, and helping them become successful adults is very important.

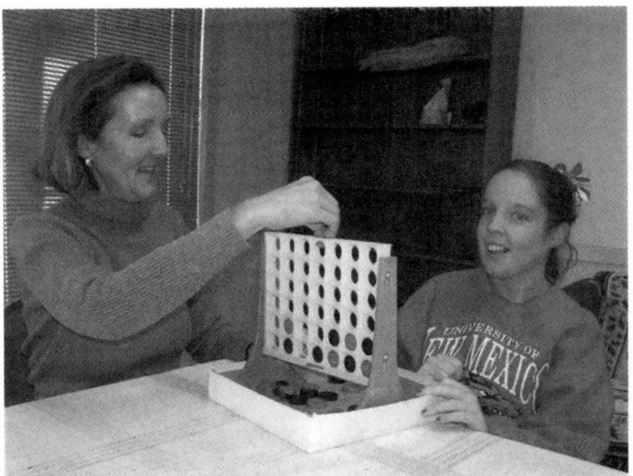

"You are the best advocate for your child, so don't let others push you into making a decision for your child that you know is not the right thing."

Sarah & Braxton

Washington

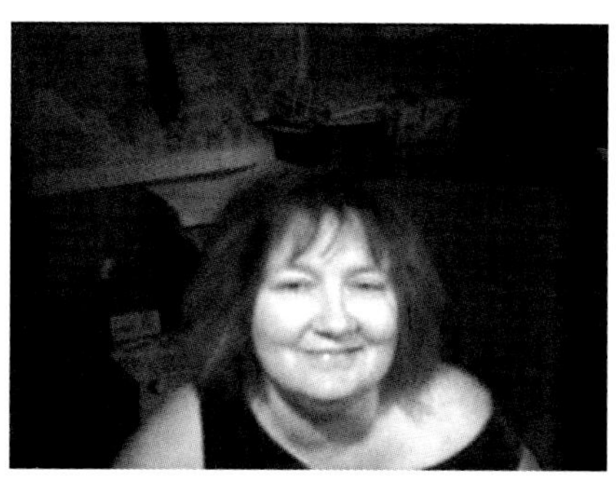

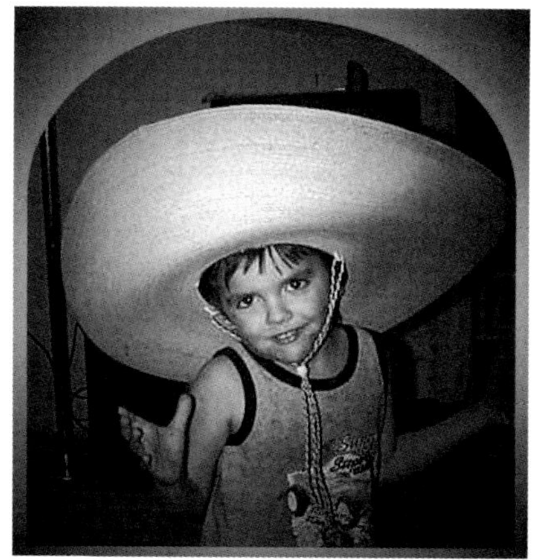

Braxton 4 years old

Braxton was diagnosed at 2 years

CONTACT:
mom2braxton@hotmail.com
www.geocities.com/mom2braxton

BIGGEST CHALLENGE(S)

My biggest challenge at this time is seeing to it that my son is educated. It seems that this school district does not want to do anything and my fear is that he will be lost in the system. He is 4 years old now and I feel strongly that what is done for him between now and 6 years old is very crucial.

Other challenges I face include being able to understand his way of communicating to me. He can't tell me he is sick or hurts. I also worry about what the future will bring for him in way of friends, etc.

Greatest Blessings

I am so blessed to have my son in my life. My little guy has taught me so much. Through him, I can see the blessings and joys in the small things such as accomplishments, etc. Every new thing he does, no matter how little, is a celebration. I see this little angel with all his challenges, with a smile all the time. My, how that warms my heart!

Words of Wisdom

Look at each day as a new day of opportunity. Look at the world through your child's eyes. Grab the opportunity to educate others on autism and let them see the blessings you have.

The 'experts' saw a child in a "world of his own"..
I see the brightest ray of sunshine.
They saw a child who "may never speak"..
I see a gift that needs no words.
They saw a child with "limited possibility"..
I see a child, my child, who can soar past the heavens.

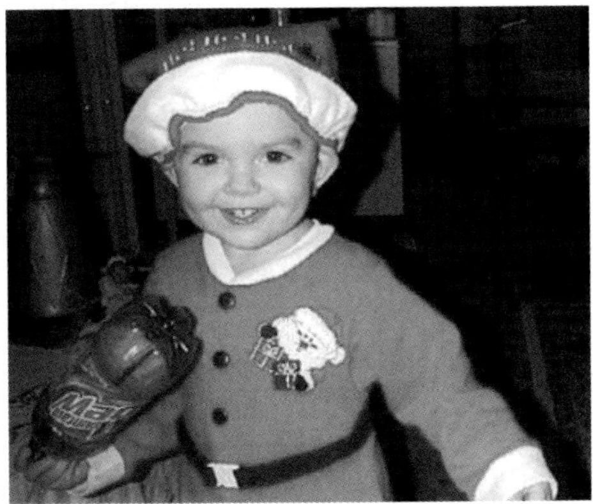

Braxton18 months

The 'experts' saw a child in a "world of his own"...
I see the brightest ray of sunshine.
They saw a child who "may never speak"...
I see a gift that needs no words.
They saw a child with "limited possibility"...
I see a child, my child,
who can soar past the heavens.

Sharon & Austin

Kansas

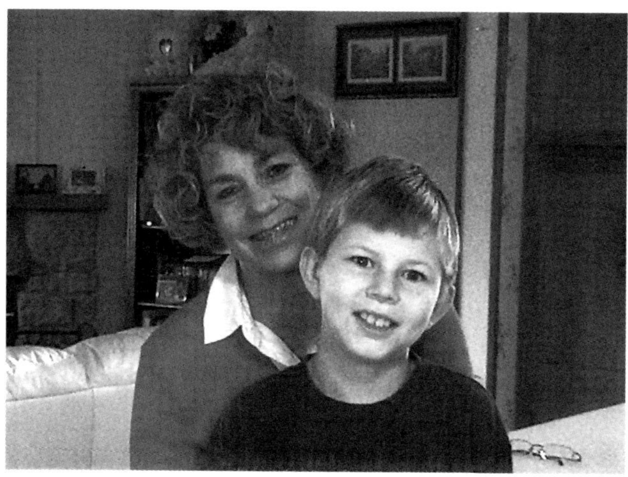

CONTACT:
mccartertexas@yahoo.com

Austin was diagnosed at 5 years

BIGGEST CHALLENGE(S)

When Austin was first diagnosed with PDD-NOS (Pervasive Developmental Disorder-not Otherwise Specified) and we were shown where it fits in the autism spectrum, we were handed a stack of papers and told, "Good luck!" It was pretty overwhelming! Luckily, I work in the medical field and have a friend that works in the mental health field; she suggested a psychiatrist that specializes in working with children with autism. From there it was like putting a very difficult puzzle together in trying to find out how we could help him and what services were available. This was especially difficult when the disability changed constantly. We were totally naive to what was coming and what to expect. He is 12-years-old now, we've been down a lot of different avenues and are still finding new ways to help him, but only by trial and error.

Secondly, we live in a rural community. A major struggle has been what seems to be the lack of educational understanding of the autism spectrum and how different it can look in each person, hence pervasive. We were not aware of our rights as advocates for our son and so in the process have lost some very important years of education for him. We continue to educate ourselves and encourage the need for educating the staff who are working with people with autism.

Greatest Blessings

We've have raised two wonderful sons already! Austin's brothers are 21 and 23. We've already been through the preteen and teen years with them and survived, so we know what that looks like. Even though Austin is 12 – that fun preteen 'I know more than you' stage – he's really not there. He is for the most part, the most loving boy. His family is the most important thing in his life.

Christ is the center part of our lives and whether Austin understands or not, He has become important for Austin as well. We pray daily and if we forget to, he promptly reminds us. One day he and I were walking to a local store near my work, we saw a young man that I would see often hanging out at a local coffee house. I always speak to the young man, that day Austin said to me after we had passed the young man with greetings, "Mom next time give him money!" I ask him why? He said "Because we are Christians!" Further questioning Austin, I discovered he thought the man was homeless since he was hanging out and he had tattered clothes. I thought "and this is a person that isn't supposed to understand the social communications of the world!" This made me laugh!

Austin has taught us patience and not to take things for granted, such as reading, writing, and just every day things we feel and see.

Words of Wisdom

- Your child is your child first, not a disability.
- Early intervention, early intervention, early intervention...
- You are your child's best advocate, you know him best.
- Never take no as an answer from the school system if there is something you think will help your child. Find ways to help them make it work for them and him, if possible.
- Never feel bad about looking down dead-end roads, at least you are trying.
- Educate yourself on the disability.
- Medication may or may not be right for your child. Weigh your options, side effects and give it some time if you decide to try it for your child. Like everything else your child is unique, they have to find the drug that is right for your child. We went through some zombie stages, picking stages, etc., until we found what worked for Austin. He has been on the same medications for 1½ years and doing great! He will tell you it makes him feel in control, so that is important to us how it makes him feel, not just us and our convenience.

One of the best things we've done as parents is to get involved in support groups, parent networking, seminars, etc. It's so nice to know you're not alone. We've found new ideas and suggestions from other parents. When you feel life can't get any harder, look at someone else's hardships. Sometimes when we get so caught up in what's going on, we forget to laugh at ourselves and to laugh at the situation. It is healthy to laugh! We've laughed and cried with other parents when talking about the things our kids do.

Favorite Resources:

1) *Thinking In Pictures*, By Temple Grandin
2) *The Out of Sync Child*, By Carol Stock Kranowitz, M.A.

Sheri & David

Kansas

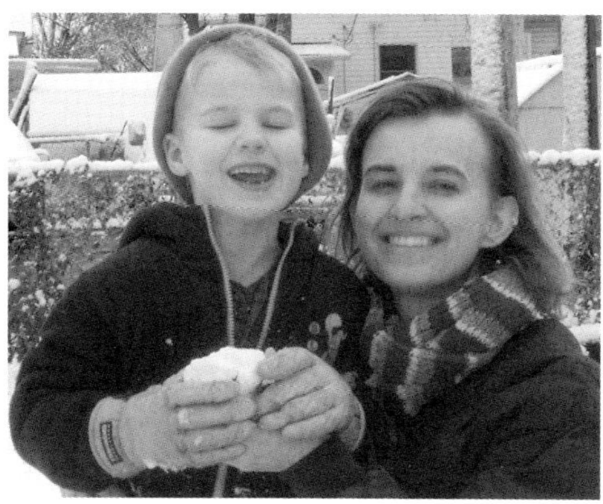

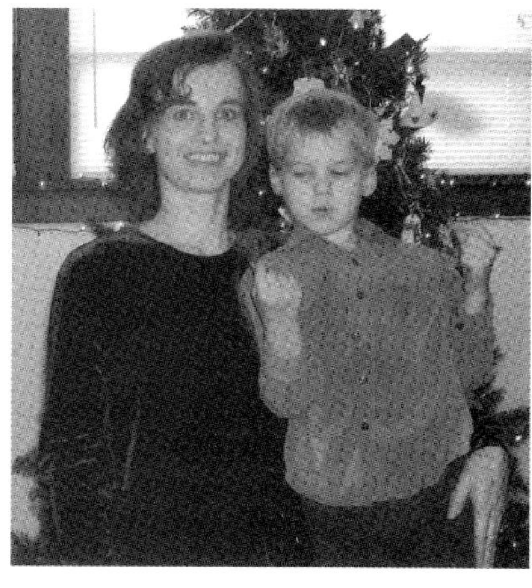

Contact:

sherifmoore@hotmail.com

David was diagnosed at 4½ years

Biggest Challenge(s)

After initiating help for my son's limited verbal exchange at age 3, ECSE. evaluation led to knowledge, acceptance, and ongoing awareness of sensory integration, expressive and receptive communication, cognitive information processing, and everything related to autism. (PDD-NOS diagnosis was at age 4½). Becoming proficient within the educational and governmental and intervention systems intended for support has continued to demand my attention and limit hobbies. These systems include school services and IEPs; Medicaid and SRS; special education law; church, family, and neighbor relations; family support grant; case management; advocacy, and biological interventions.

Learning about normal age level developmental milestones and helping my son understand, respond and attain those goals is requiring extra research in the various categories of his needs. It is like trying to learn the functions behind what speech therapists, occupational therapists, and special education teachers do and then trying to work with that information confidently, without a degree, certificate or salary. It is easy for me to feel discouraged and frustrated when my son responds with inattention or resistance. I also feel unaccomplished and incomplete at my parent/teacher role when play and purposeful learning times together are not progressing as I would like.

I intensely desire to complete the Defeat Autism Now biological testing and also to implement the Relationship Development Intervention therapy (www.R.D.I.com), but lack the financial resources. So I am frustrated by limited support and limited use of potentially benefiting treatment.

And I miss being in friendships and relationships that are not entwined emotionally with the role of my dominance or concerns over something related to my child's needs. I tire of explaining things about autism, David's levels of needs and interaction, cooking and eating within the CFGF diet, potty training, and making teachers and helpers uncomfortable. I fear I have joined my child in becoming "out of sync" (but recognize I cannot be in sync with everyone).

Greatest Blessings

The most exciting blessings that keep me going come from the exchange of prayers and answers from God. He provided a basement area educational room in our new home at my request to home educate. He has opened my mind to understand more about autism, how to communicate effectively, and how to model speech and promote developmental age skills with my younger children at home and at church. He has given us a welcoming and effective children's ministry department at our church. He has helped us grow through using the services of various dedicated public school special education staff and private speech and preschool services. He has given me a mentoring family in my city with similar outlook and advanced experience with autism. He has enabled us to find and receive help through the information and contacts with others dealing with similar needs, including our monthly support group meetings at Topeka Autism and Asperger Resource Center. He has allowed us to receive government financial assistance through S.S.I., family support grant, and Medicaid.

My vision for my son's future is proactive and positive to accept his worth and value, regardless of exact occupation or ministry involvement. That gives me some fulfillment too. I have an increased motivation and sense of fulfillment to "share the wealth" in improving my state of being by finding financial, emotional, physical and spiritual resources. It looks like I will indefinitely keep praying, researching, and implementing in this management position called motherhood, but supposedly willingly and with a pleasant disposition. So help me God.

Words of Wisdom

My pep talk: Go for the "master's degree" in mothering an autistic child. Keep aware of interacting with your child as more important than rotely performing the therapies themselves. If you have doubts, needs or concerns – ask God about it and find others to help. Don't give up. Keep trying to understand more, take responsibility, and know that nobody can surpass the potential impact of benefit for your child as well as you. God made you your child's mother, and God can sustain you and your child.

Stacey & Erin

Alaska

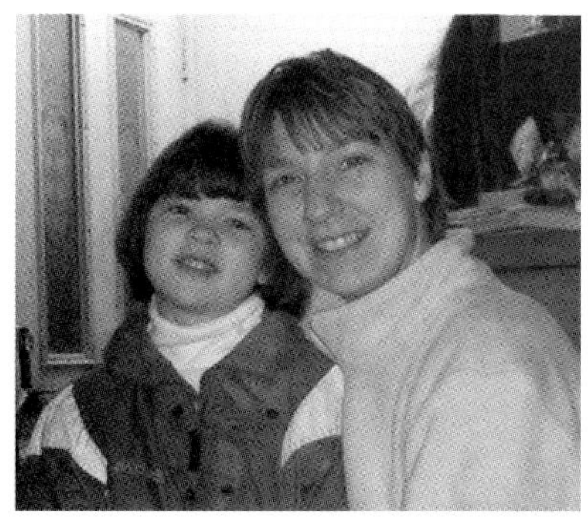

Erin age 5

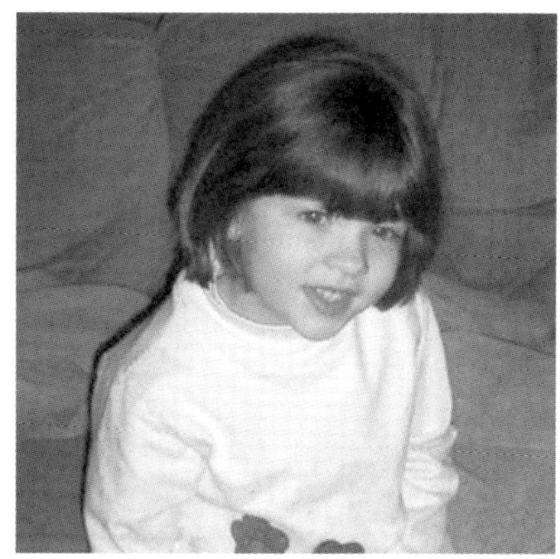

Erin was diagnosed at 4 years

Contact:

lanes907@hotmail.com

Biggest Challenge(s)

Our biggest challenge was our first year starting Dietary Intervention and going gluten (wheat), casein (dairy), and soy free. We faced a lot of skepticism from our friends, family, and doctors in those first few months. I spent a lot of time trying to educate people about it, only to find they still looked at me like I was some crazed parent trying to "cure" my child. That is, until Erin started to emerge from the confines of autism. Within a month, the "brain fog" began to lift. She started facing us and looking into our eyes instead of looking at our eyes for a fleeting moment. Her communication skills surpassed my greatest hopes when she started to talk spontaneously without prompts. It has now been two years since implementing the GFCF diet and she has gained over 3 years of language. It still amazes me that food intolerances play such a huge role in her behavior, sleep patterns, and ability to learn. I only wish we knew about this five years ago. All in all, our biggest challenge has become our most gratifying reward.

Greatest Blessings

When Erin was a toddler, we would take long walks in our small seaside town. I was always in a hurry to get from Point A to Point B. Erin on the other hand always wanted to stop and smell the flowers...literally. I remember trying to hurry her up although there was no reason to be in a rush. One day it just occurred to me...slow down and enjoy the moment. Now we enjoy and appreciate the small things in life. The flowers, the feel of raindrops on our faces, a shared smile when she sees that "Mommy's getting 'the big picture'". She is my Greatest Blessing and it's moments like these that make me realize in many ways she is the teacher, and I the student.

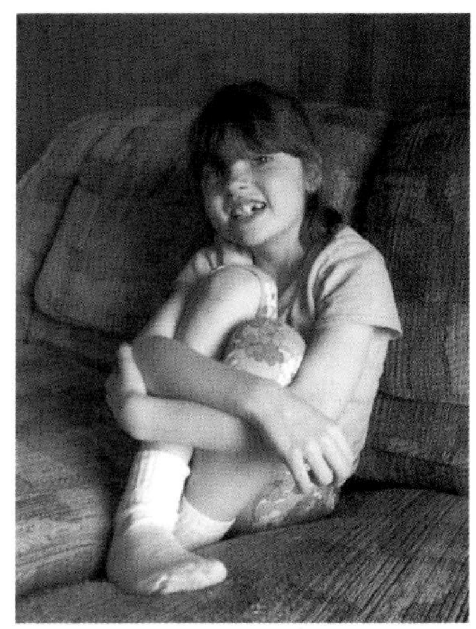

Erin 7 years old

Words of Wisdom

Think outside of the box and follow your instincts. If I had listened to every person that said "That won't work!", I may never have heard her say "I love you!"

Favorite Resources:

1) *Special Diets for Special Kids* (book one and two) by Lisa Lewis PhD
2) *Unraveling the Mysteries of Autism and Pervasive Developmental Disorder* by Karyn Seroussi
3) *Laughing & Loving with Autism* (there's about 3 of them)
4) Future Horizons Website http://futurehorizons-autism.com
5) The Autism Research Institute www.autism.com/ari
6) The GFCF Diet website www.gfcfdiet.com
7) Support organization in Alaska www.stonesoupgroup.org (just opened up a Family-to-Family Health Information Center for families caring for children with special health care needs!)

"Think outside of the box and follow your instincts. If I had listened to every person that said 'That won't work!', I may never have heard her say 'I love you!'"

Sue & Tyler

Illinois

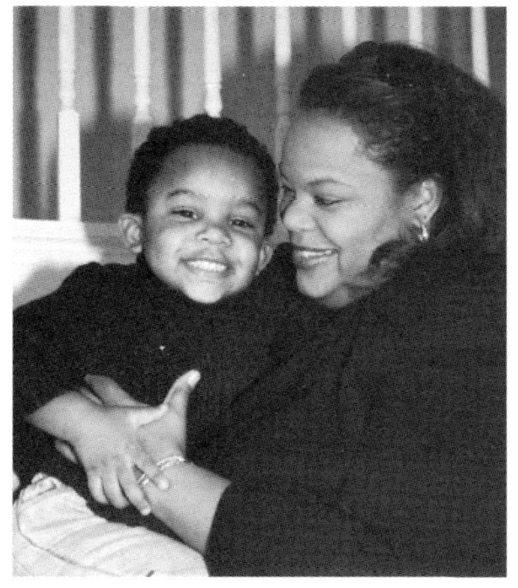

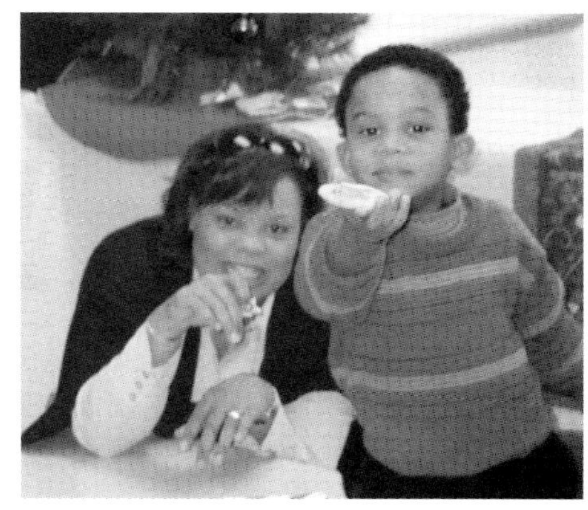

Tyler was diagnosed PDD at 4 years

CONTACT:
suebw@comcast.net

BIGGEST CHALLENGE(S)

Fear of the unknown is one of my greatest challenges. Will Tyler be able to function as an adult? Will he marry and have children? Will he lead a "normal" life? You really have to take it one year at a time. He makes such great strides every year that I am afraid it will all end and that one year he may just stall. Doctors are no help in this department because they always give the routine response of "every child is different."

Also, trying to explain Tyler's PDD to friends or even family is difficult. Because Tyler can speak and is social, people often think I'm over exaggerating his condition. They say, "Oh, he's fine. Those doctors don't know what they're talking about." Then you notice them staring at him because he can't respond to their questions or he sits through the entire circus with his ears covered because he will become over stimulated. It takes a family with incredible patience to deal with an autistic child.

Greatest Blessings

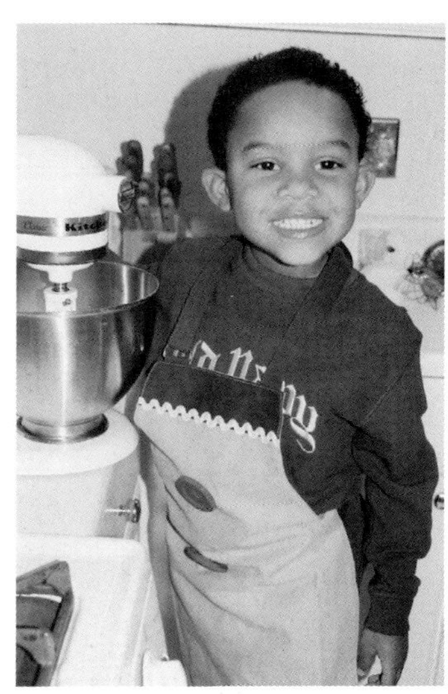

I am so blessed to have a great support group. My parents are Tyler's nannies and they take their job very seriously. They attend all his functions and some doctor appointments and asked for reports from the doctors!

Tyler is also blessed with attending a pre-school filled with teachers who love and care for him. Tyler's first year of pre-school was spent in a class specifically geared toward children with autism. He blossomed so quickly with the more structured lesson plan he was able to transition into a "traditional class." This year, at age 5, Tyler is in a typical class with typical children and progressing very well. He is able to look to those children as role models and what is so wonderful is THEY see Tyler as just another classmate. Tyler and the other special needs children are treated just like anyone else in the class.

Words of Wisdom

Count your blessings for what your child CAN do! Do not become discouraged by what he/she is not able to do... it may come.

Treat your autistic child just like you would treat a "typical kid." Let him/her run, jump and play... let them enjoy their freedoms as a child. Be grateful for every progression and milestone your child makes. Listen to your doctors but pray for your child's progression as well! And finally, be your child's advocate for the care and instruction he/she is entitled to. If you don't stand up for your own child who will?

> "Count your blessings for what your child CAN do! Do not become discouraged by what he/she is not able to do... it may come."

Sue & Tyler

Wisconsin

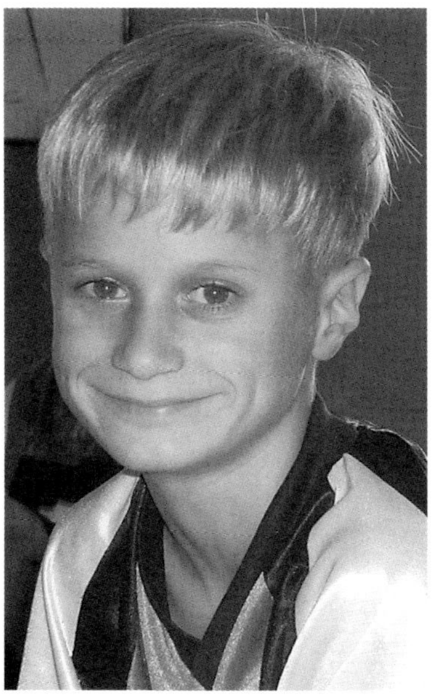

CONTACT:
sgwcri@aol.com

Tyler was diagnosed at 5 years

BIGGEST CHALLENGE(S)

Every day can be a roller coaster ride. I don't know if the day will be uphill or downhill, fast moving, or nice and steady. Sometimes, people will look at us with a frightful glare or a friendly smile. They don't "see" my son's disability. He's not in a wheel chair or walking with crutches. He looks "normal" but doesn't always act it. My biggest fear is that kids will bully him and he won't understand. If I could only help him make one good friend through his journey of life...

Greatest Blessings

Tyler sees life as simple. Things usually don't bother him like they bother us. He is the most caring child and will share anything of his. He has faith in God like no other. He let's balloons go – just to give them to Jesus!

Words of Wisdom

God made no mistake by giving you this child. He/she is yours for a reason. He gave you only what you can handle – and you can handle this precious gift!

> He has faith in God like no other.
> He let's balloons go
> – just to give them to Jesus!

Susan & Jake

North Carolina

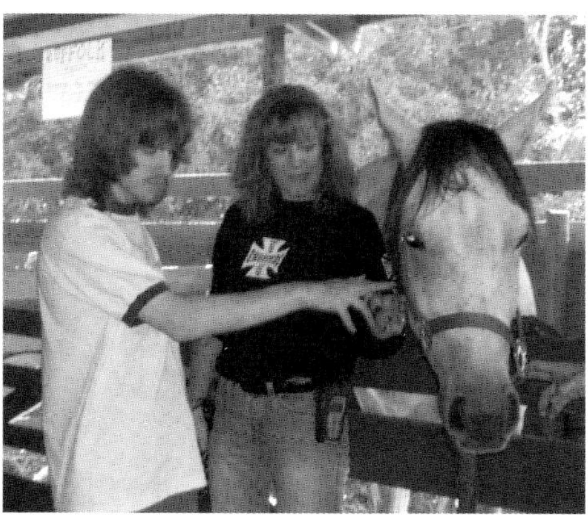

Jake was diagnosed at 18 months

Biggest Challenge(s)

- I would LOVE to have a conversation with my son. I have always wondered what he is thinking.
- It hurts to have never heard him call me "Mama".
- He is in a group home. Sometimes I feel like everyone else has forgot about him but me.
- Seeing kids his age and thinking about what he would be doing if he was "normal". It breaks my heart.
- Having to put him in a group home was the hardest thing I have ever done in my whole life.
- Taking him out in public and having to deal with rude people.
- The constant fight to have proper care for him.
- The day he was diagnosed with severe autism. It was like the death of the son I thought I had and a new world I had to enter that I didn't want to be.

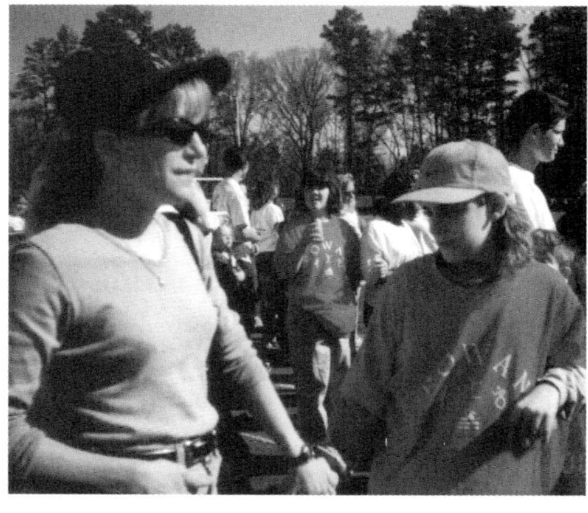

Greatest Blessings

- When he learns something new, even if it is something he should have done years ago, I am thrilled he can do it now.
- When he smiles at me.
- To look at how beautiful he is.
- When he really looks me in the eyes.
- A kiss from him.
- When someone remembers him and asks me "how is Jake?"
- That he is alive and I have the joy of being his Mom.
- That he is usually happy. I want him to enjoy his life.

Words of Wisdom

- Never give up on anything that pertains to your child.
- Fight for what you want.
- Your heart and instincts know what is best for your child.
- Try not to let other people's stupid remarks hurt your feelings.
- Try not to let their behavior in public embarrass you. Tell yourself "it doesn't matter what other people think".
- Love them just for being them.

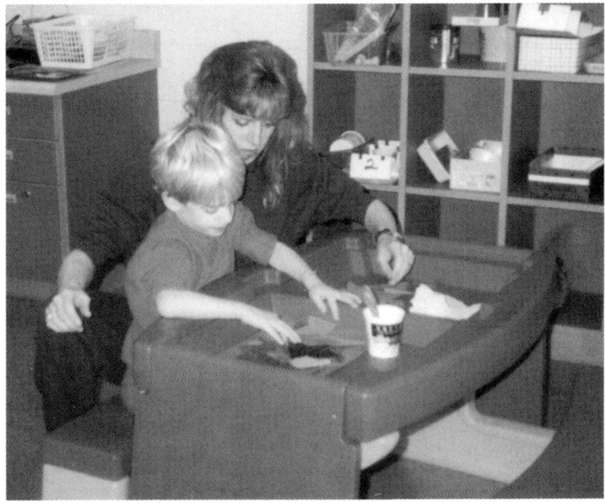

Susie & Ryan

Missouri

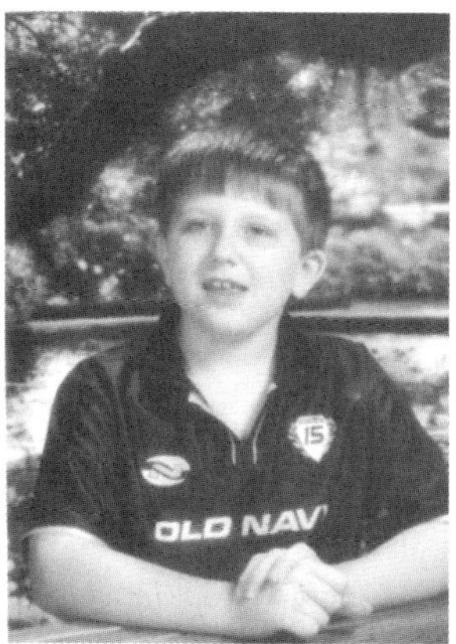

CONTACT:
mopar1@centurytel.net

Ryan was diagnosed at 19 months

BIGGEST CHALLENGE & GREATEST BLESSING

Our biggest challenge I believe is to read about and understand autism and use that knowledge to help our son live normal as a life as possible. Their needs to be change and the search for knowledge is never-ending. Applying it and seeing results would be the greatest blessing. Plus, knowing that God has given us the blessing of a child that is always loving and understanding inspires us to do the best we can. Our child is not aggressive and is always wanting to work hard and to please us.

WORDS OF WISDOM

The wisdom comes with time and patience. These children help us to appreciate the little, simple things.

This is a poem written for Ryan when he was first diagnosed – I entered it in an American Mothers Contest and received first place. I dedicated it to all mothers with disabled children. - *Susie*

Life with Autism

You might have heard the word and wondered such as I,
What this disorder consisted of and why?
Why the brain could only work in such a way,
To make life so complex each and every day.
With proper understanding, training, and trust,
You all learn to cope and see living is a must!
To make it into "their world" is worth the time,
You see things their way – you understand their mind,
They are very individual, that point is clear,
But they love our love and being held near.
Their way of showing this may appear odd
But all it takes to see may be a simple nod.
When life is broken down to the most precious of things,
These children are there; they are God's special beings.
We must love them, be there, share smallest of imperfections,
They have been given to us to lead us in the 'right' direction.

Tera & Kaeden

Belgium

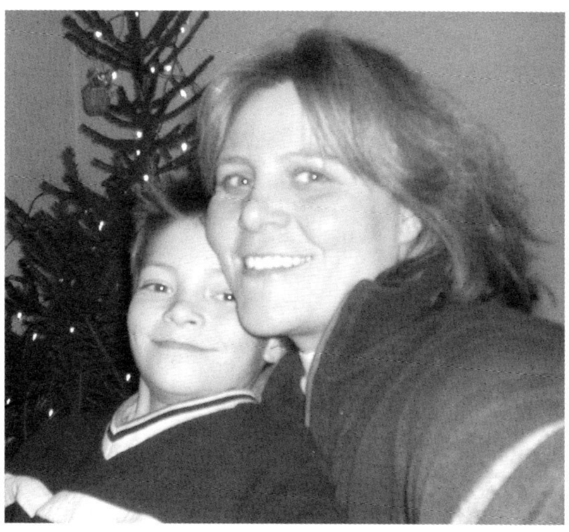

CONTACT:

christer@tiscali.be

Kaeden was diagnosed at 8 years

BIGGEST CHALLENGE(S)

Autism – such a small word that creates such panic within my soul. I hear it, I think it, I breathe it, I research it, I explain it, I dream it, I live it, and yet, to this day, I have no idea what it precisely is. What I do know is that my son, Kaeden, has this disorder that creates havok in our home and our lives as we try to get a grasp on how to deal with this little word, autism.

How do I deal with autistic behavior? And when exactly is my son exhibiting autistic behavior and when is he simply being a brat that needs reprimanded? This is my biggest challenge in dealing with autism. I simply do not know how to read him. As our day goes along and everything seems so normal, one simple word or question or gesture could set him off and the peace that reigned our home only minutes before becomes a battle zone, each family member on a different team with his own game plan. Unfortunately, nobody ever wins the war and we each crawl away with battle scars that leave pain on our hearts.

The "behaviors" Kaeden acts out are typical of what any naughty kid would do. He hits, he curses, he is disrespectful and doesn't listen. The problem is that sometimes he does these things without himself realizing he is doing them. He doesn't mean to be naughty, his world just overtakes him and living in ours becomes too great a chore. And yet, other times, he truly is being a normal kid that has to learn right from wrong, and as his mother it is my job to teach him. I want my son to grow up to live as a productive member of society. But how can I do this when sometimes he is not even living in the same world as I am? How do I know when to just let it go and when to make it a learning moment? Learning to read Kaeden is a great challenge, but I am a determined mama, and I will keep crawling away from each battle with a bit more knowledge to help me overcome this challenge of autism. I still have no answers, only questions that I try to answer 24 hours/day, 7 days/week. How do I tackle this little boy that I want to make into a man?

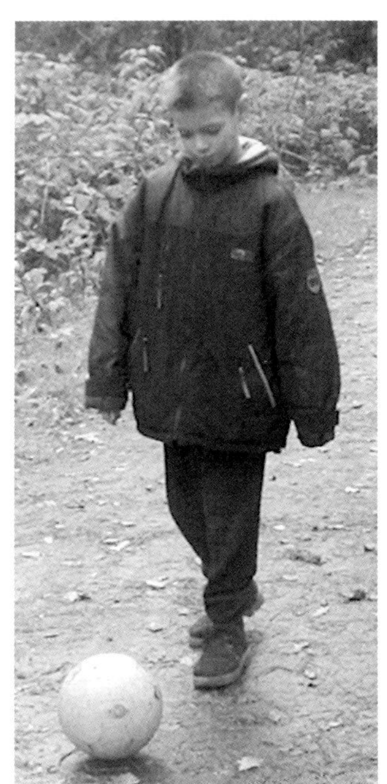

Greatest Blessings

When I think back to the early years with my son as a single mother, I know that the greatest blessing in our lives has been my husband, Erwin. He came into our lives when Kaeden was three with expectations of a happy family and no preview of what was to come. He has stood by our side through thousands of "appointments" ranging from psychiatrist, school, doctor, therapy, video training, autism society, etc. The shock of reality with Kaeden creates so much additional stress, anger, and confusion in an already compound situation as we unite into a family. It has been an ongoing battle, yet my husband, Kaeden's papa, continues to kiss us each night before we go to sleep, assure us everything will be okay, and give us the love and support we need. He may not always react in the manner I find suited to the situation, but he is doing what he feels is best for us, and he has not wavered in his dedication to us or our family. He also shared in bringing Jari, our youngest son, into our family. Jari is the greatest gift I have ever and will ever give Kaeden. He loves his baby brother to the end of the earth and back. When I pray and thank God each night before I close my eyes for all the gifts in my life, I can't help but know I have been blessed; my life is so rich with all the love surrounding me from my three guys. For Kaeden, Erwin has become a security and comfort, the man he looks up to and learns from. Yes, the greatest blessing for both of us.

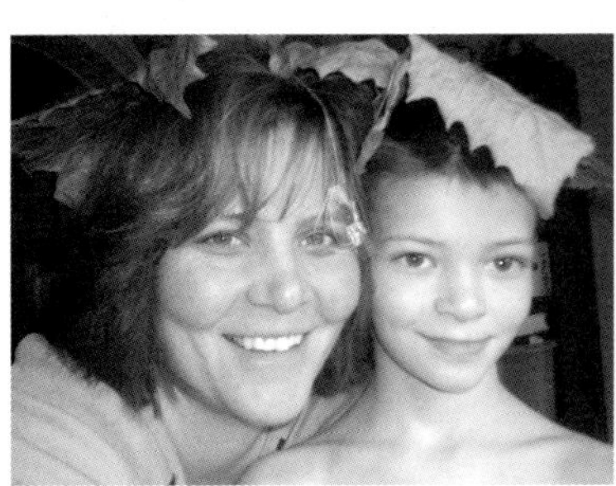

Words of Wisdom

What I know about parenting a child with autism is that God chose me for this job. He chose me for a reason and He never gives more than you can handle. When I look at my son and fear overwhelms me, I only have to glance his way again and feel the love that flows through me and I know it will be okay (I can say this today, but maybe tomorrow is another story completely. Living with an autistic child is such a life of change…you have to be ready for anything). Through all the tears and tribulations, pain and miscommunication, there is something greater. My Kaeden is a little boy who loves to laugh and play and be proud. He speaks to me more deeply than any other person in the world. He gives me so much hope in one small moment that no one else would consider noteworthy. Each day when I wake and see my early riser I know the sun is shining before I even look outside. Kaeden is that shimmer that brings light to my life. When I discovered I was going to be a mommy, I had no idea what I was in for. I continue to learn and I continue to do my best to be happy and successful and raise my children to do and be the same. Whether Kaeden was autistic or not, my goal is still the same. It puts a twist on the reality of everyday life, but the goal hasn't changed…I want to be a mama that my son will stand up proudly and say to all the world "Look there, that is MY mom." And when I look deep into his eyes I can see that he is content and happy. I continue to have hope.

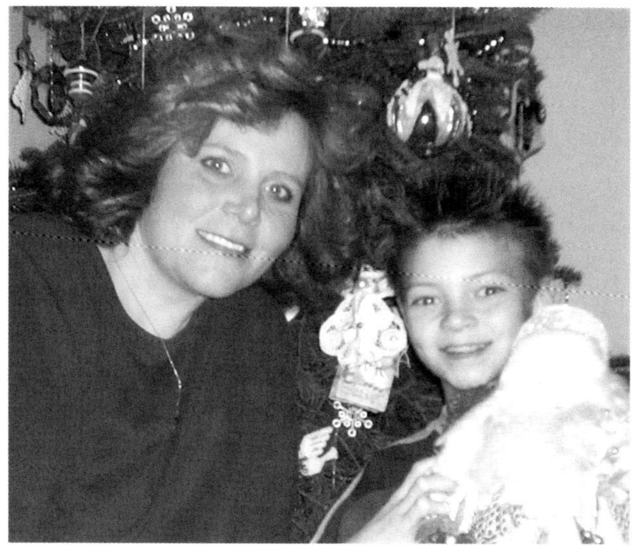

Autism/Asperger's/PDD

In an effort to 'fill' this extra page – I decided to list the definition of the Autism Spectrum for those who are not familiar with it. This was taken from NICHCY (National Dissemination Center for Children with Disabilities.) Due to space limitations, only a portion of the definitions are reprinted here so please visit www.NICHCY.org for a more complete description.

Also, I personally prefer that my daughter is referred to as 'having autism' rather than 'being autistic'. — *Judy*

Autistic Disorder, sometimes referred to as early infantile autism or childhood autism, is four times more common in boys than in girls. Children with Autistic Disorder have a moderate to severe range of communication, socialization, and behavior problems. Many children with autism also have mental retardation.

Asperger's Disorder, also referred to as Asperger's or Asperger's Syndrome, is a developmental disorder characterized by a lack of social skills; difficulty with social relationships; poor coordination and poor concentration; and a restricted range of interests, but normal intelligence and adequate language skills in the areas of vocabulary and grammar. Asperger's Disorder appears to have a somewhat later onset than Autistic Disorder, or at least is recognized later. An individual with Asperger's Disorder does not possess a significant delay in language development; however, he or she may have difficulty understanding the subtleties used in conversation, such as irony and humor. Also, while many individuals with autism have mental retardation, a person with Asperger's possesses an average to above average intelligence (Autism Society of America, 1995). Asperger's is sometimes incorrectly referred to as "high-functioning autism."

Pervasive Developmental Disorder Not Otherwise Specified (PDD-NOS)
Generally, an individual is diagnosed as having PDDNOS if he or she has some behaviors that are seen in autism but does not meet the full DSM-IV criteria for having Autistic Disorder. Despite the DSM-IV concept of Autistic Disorder and PDDNOS being two distinct types of PDD, there is clinical evidence suggesting that Autistic Disorder and PDDNOS are on a continuum (i.e., an individual with Autistic Disorder can improve and be rediagnosed as having PDDNOS, or a young child can begin with PDDNOS, develop more autistic features, and be rediagnosed as having Autistic Disorder). For a more complete description, see www.NICHCY.org

Teresa & Nick

Oklahoma

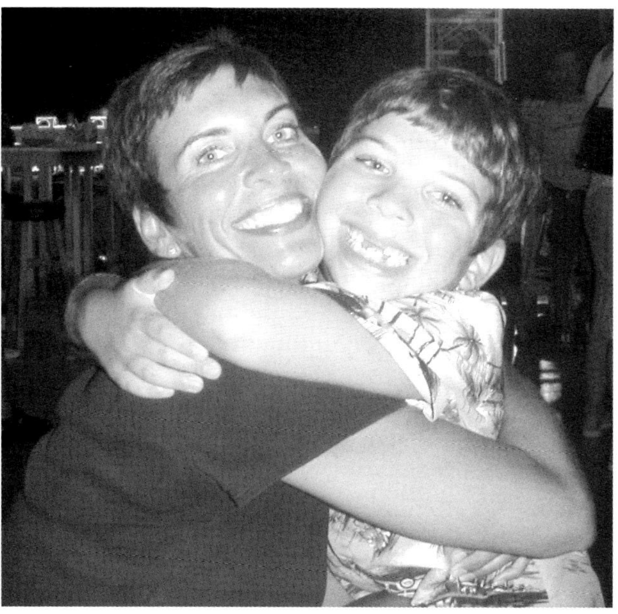

Nick 8 years old

CONTACT:
tlwaters@swbell.net
580-223-5013

Nick was diagnosed PDD/NOS at 18 months

BIGGEST CHALLENGE(S)

- Grieving for the loss of the child I thought I had.
- Accepting that the future is unknown.
- Trying everything I could to help my son. Every treatment that I heard or read about, I tried. Some were so hard to put him through.
- Having to admit that some of the treatments were not effective, when you wanted to say you could see a change, but actually there was none.
- Watching him in the beginning of his ABA therapy cry until he would fall asleep on the floor during the session.

Greatest Blessings

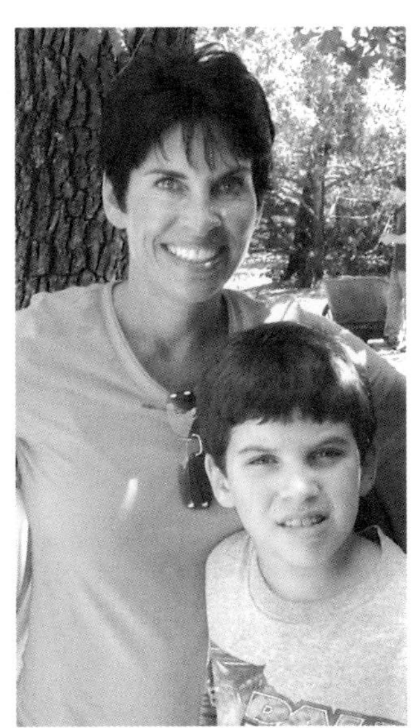

- Nick has brought up more blessings than I could list. We have many wonderful people in our lives because of his autism.
- His brothers have a compassion for others, well beyond their years.
- Watching Nick accomplish things, big and small. Some things we never gave a second thought to with his older brothers.
- Learning to look at people's abilities instead of their inabilities.

Words of Wisdom

- Grieve when you feel the need. I still have periods of grief, and my son is doing great. There is still a sense of loss from time to time.
- The unknown future has brought many good things. All of the things I feared Nick would never do, he has accomplished, i.e., talking, understanding, riding a bike, potty training, tying his own shoes, and going to a regular school.
- Don't be afraid to ask others for help.
- Never be ashamed of autism. It is a part, and only a part, of your child.
- Raise your expectations of your child. You'll be surprised how they will arise to the occasion.
- Never give up. I believe that our children can always learn and improve.
- I thank God for autism when I hear of families with children who are dying. There are a lot of deadly diseases out there, but autism is not one of them!
- Take care of yourself so that you can take care of your child.
- You did not cause your child's autism. Do not blame yourself.

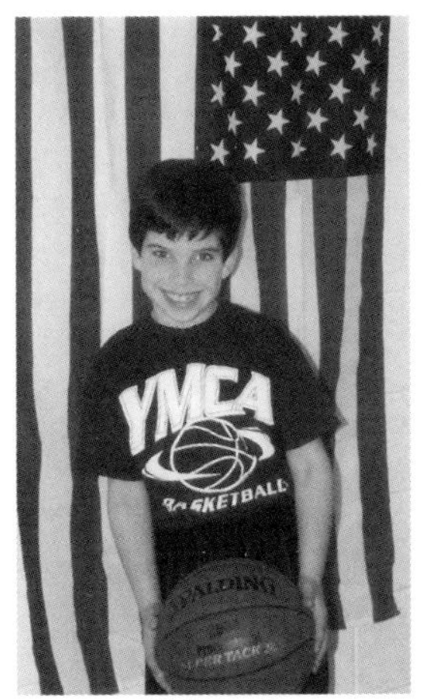

Nick age 8

"Raise your expectations of your child. You'll be surprised how they will arise to the occasion."

Terry & Kurt

Missouri

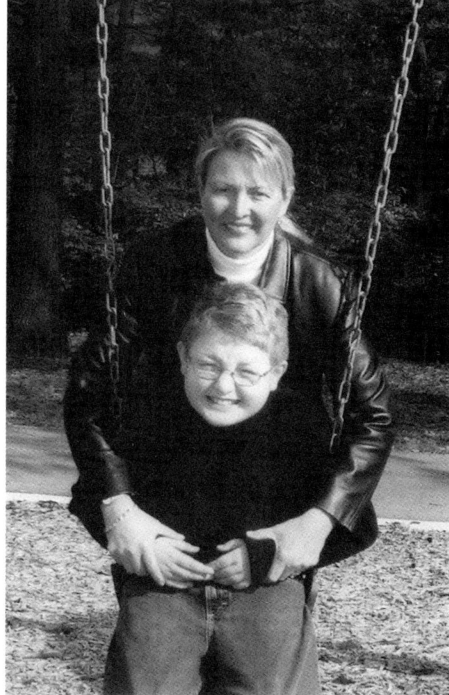

Kurt was diagnosed at 27 months

CONTACT:
mjmtam@aol.com

Nine years ago my life took a different direction, my youngest son Kurt was born and twenty-seven months later he was diagnosed with autism. This was not the end of my world, but the beginning of a journey in a different world. Kurt has made me a different person. I live my life one day at a time and have learned not to sweat the small stuff. He has taught me to slow down and enjoy each and every day and the joy in that day. Because of autism I have met some of the most inspiring and caring individuals. Kurt's great progress is because of the love of family, friends, and some of the most dedicated teachers, classmates, and therapists out there. But mostly, I thank God for entrusting the care of this beautiful angel to me! My world would not be complete without the continued love and support of my husband Mike and my oldest son, and Kurt's best friend, his brother Brett.

"He has taught me to slow down and enjoy each and every day and the joy in that day."

Favorite Resources and Recommendations:

1) ABA (Applied Behavior Analysis)
2) Kirkman Labs has great vitamin supplements for children/adults with autism. They have a catalog. Kirkmanlabs.com.
3) Get this book....*Biological Treatment for Autism and PDD* by W. Shaw, Ph. D
4) PECS (Picture Exchange Communication) This is an awesome form of communication for children that are non-verbal.
5) DIET: Many individuals with autism benefit from a gluten (wheat) and casein free diet (dairy). Limit sugars and food dyes too!
6) Tag on shoe. If a child has difficulty communicating, I recommend a tag on their shoelace with name and phone number. (Petsmart has a machine to make one up quickly.)
7) Swim and Walk...lots of physical exercise.
8) Trampoline (small exercise ones can usually be found at garage sales for a few dollars).
9) Music: Always play music at home and in the car. Get music therapy if possible, I have yet to see a child with autism not benefit from music in a positive way! Native American music seems to be popular now with kids!
10) Other suggestions...weighted vest, brushin/joint compressions. Any occupational therapist should be able to advise on these.
11) Support Groups for Parents and Siblings (maybe contact Judevine Center for Autism AND MO-FEAT).
12) Keep your child as well-groomed and nicely dressed as possible. Appearance is always a social and acceptance plus!
13) INTERNET...type in Autism and wow!!!
14) Keep a calendar journal/diary. It helps keep all interventions and appointments organized.
15) NEW THERAPY: Relationship Development Intervention (RDI) website: rdiconnect.com. This is awesome!!
16) Educate Everyone! Knowledge is Power!
17) Read current books, 1998 on (anything before 1998 I have found can be outdated information.)
18) *Children with Autism: A Parent's Guide* by Michael Powers (2000)
19) *Understanding Autism for Dummies* by Linda Rastelli (2004)

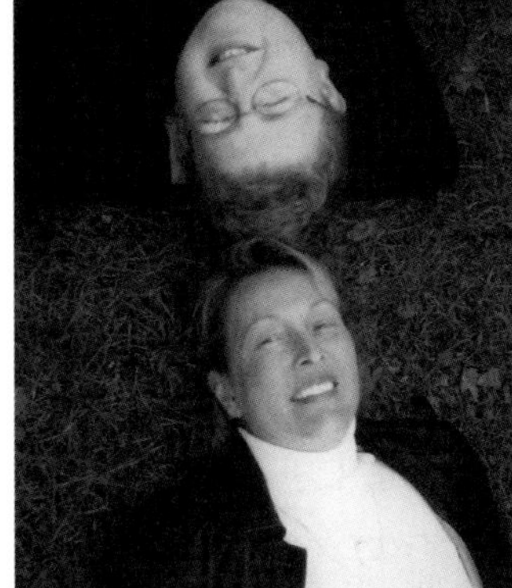

For Siblings and Schools:

20) *Joey and Sam* by Illana Katz and Edward Ritvo, M.D. (1993)
21) *My Brother Kevin Has Autism* by Richard Carlson (2002)
22) *My Friend with Autism* by Beverly Bishop (2002) (My Favorite!!)
23) *Siblings of Children with Autism: A Guide for Families* by Sandra Harris (2003)
24) *Taking Autism to School* by Andreanna Edwards (2002)

Theresa & Christina

Connecticut

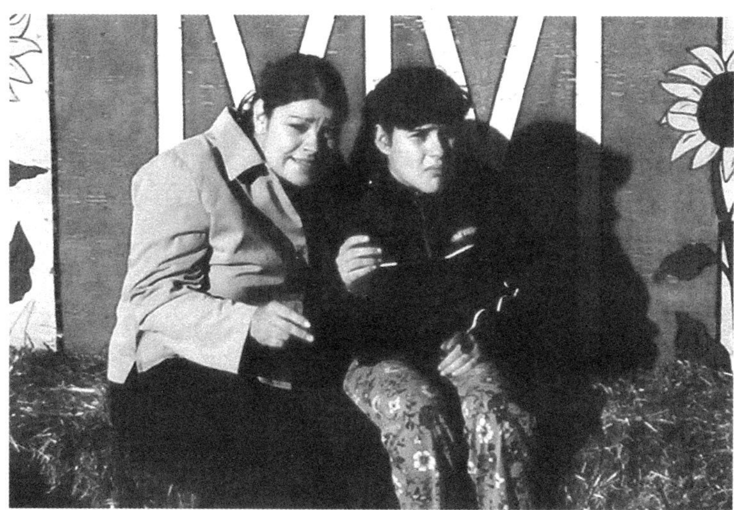

CONTACT:
tmorleslcsw@aol.com
Unlocking Autism Rep. of CT

Christina was diagnosed at 2½ years

BIGGEST CHALLENGE(S)

I honestly have to say that I have several challenges where my 12-year-old daughter, Christina, is concerned.

- I would love to be able to get a full-time job and not have to worry about who would watch my daughter. At this point, I have no one that I can trust and who is competent enough to watch Christina.
- Christina is non-verbal and it is extremely difficult when it comes to communication. It is sometimes hard to know when she feels sick or in pain unless it is really obvious.
- I have so much fear for Christina. I always fear for her safety and wonder what will happen when her dad and I pass away.
- I have trouble "letting go". I am, and always have been, overprotective. I constantly worry when Chrissy isn't with me or her dad. I worry that she may be teased, abused, or neglected. Until this past year, I've always driven her to and from school. Now she takes the school van and she is the only child with special needs. I still feel uneasy about it but I know how important it is for her to have independence.

Greatest Blessings

- Being closer to GOD
- Meeting people who have been like Godsends to us.
- My daughter has taught me so much about myself and about life.
- Realizing the depth of my character, as a person and as a mother, i.e., humility, patience, tolerance for people who don't know what having a child with autism is like, strength and appreciation for the littlest things (miracles) that Christina does.

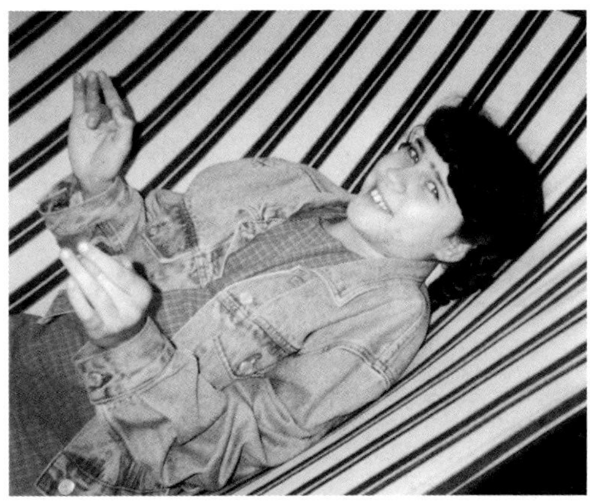

Words of Wisdom

- Believe whole-heartedly in your Faith.
- ALWAYS trust your maternal instincts/"little voice".
- Take care of yourself – you can't take care of your child if you can't take care of yourself first.
- DON'T EVER GIVE UP ON YOUR CHILD!

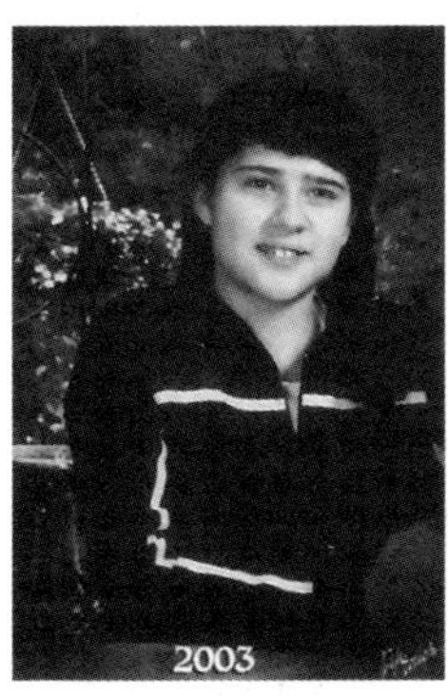

Tina, Jason & Brandon

Virginia

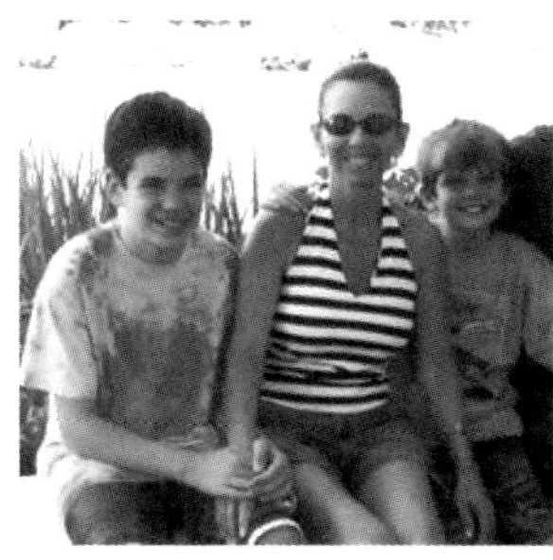

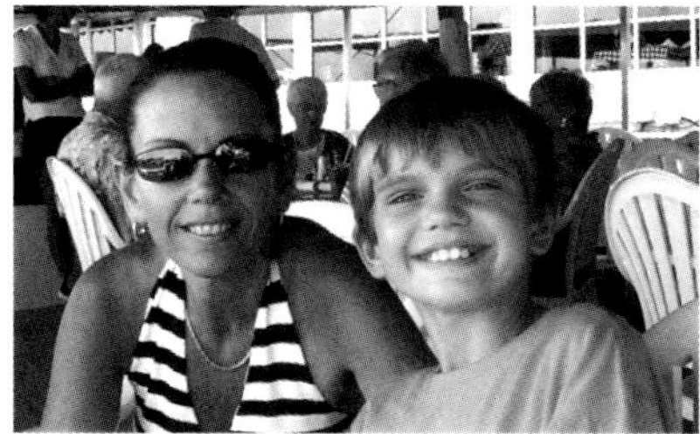

Brandon age 10

CONTACT:
fairyprincess921@adelphia.net

Jason was diagnosed at 2 years
Brandon was diagnosed at 18 months

BIGGEST CHALLENGE(S)

I am the mother of two children with special needs. Jason, who is 12, has autism, he is on the high end of the spectrum. Brandon is 10, and he has bi-polar disorder/ADHD/PDD-NOS — me, well I am 43 and diagnosed bipolar myself just 7-8 years ago. Facing all these new medical terms, learning about medications, (AND having to become an expert on them) is one challenge — wow, the list could go on. I think the day-in and day-out of continuing to love my children and myself is the hardest. I'll fight with the school for services any day, but I cringe at the thought when my children are so out of control that I have to restrain them. Jason has been in residential once, just this past September for the longest 5½ weeks of my life. I went into a major depression, but never stopped fighting until I called and got him discharged well before they felt he was ready (AMA). Brandon has been hospitalized 4 times, just came home last week from his most latest acute care stay. My biggest challenge is learning what to do to prevent these situations.

Greatest Blessings

My children. Two simple words. I love them with all my heart. They are so unique. Jason is 12 and in the "in-between" years (Oh my, I remember when he didn't even talk at age four, but could read a book at 3). Now he knows what "sexy" girls are!!!! He tries so hard, my beautiful boy, but he is so misunderstood. Having car rides with him, watching wheel of fortune, getting him to play a full board game with me, the list is endless. He is charismatic and engaging, and my angel from heaven.

Words of Wisdom

Take every day for what it is worth. Treasure the times you have now, they soon will be no more. Take pictures and videotape - they have been priceless to us. Educate your neighbors and friends and family. Do your part in taking an awareness stand. Wear your ribbons anytime, but especially during Autism Awareness Month in April. Believe in early intervention, it does work and you can watch your children grow to become productive members of your community. Reach out to people and ask them for help — do not be afraid.

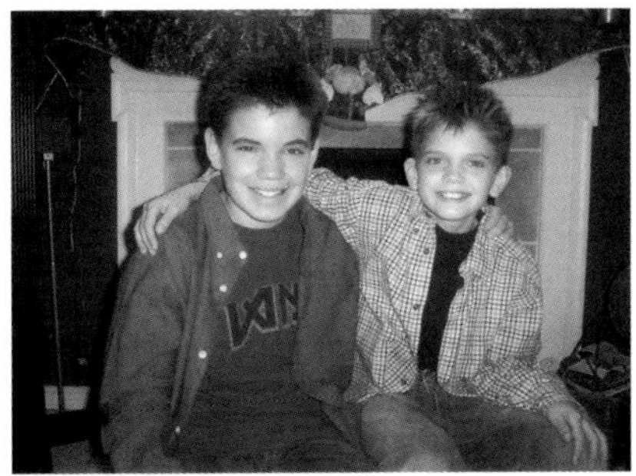

"A mother is the truest friend we have, when trials heavy and sudden, fall upon us; when friends who rejoice with us in our sunshine desert us; when trouble thickens around us, still will she cling to us, and endeavor by her kind precepts and counsels to dissipate the clouds of darkness, and cause peace to return to our hearts."

—Washington Irving

Tracy & Benjamin

Delaware

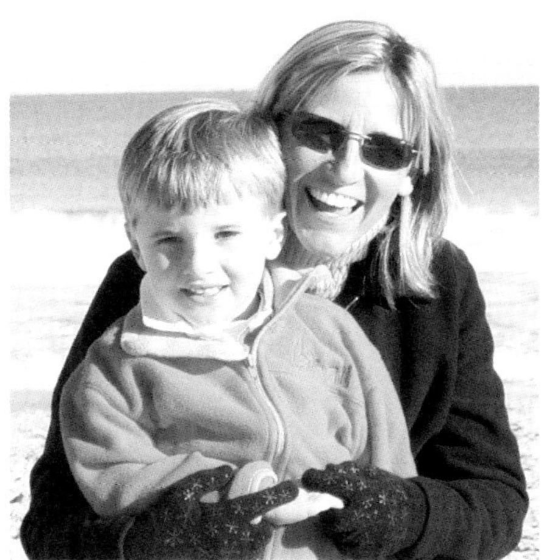

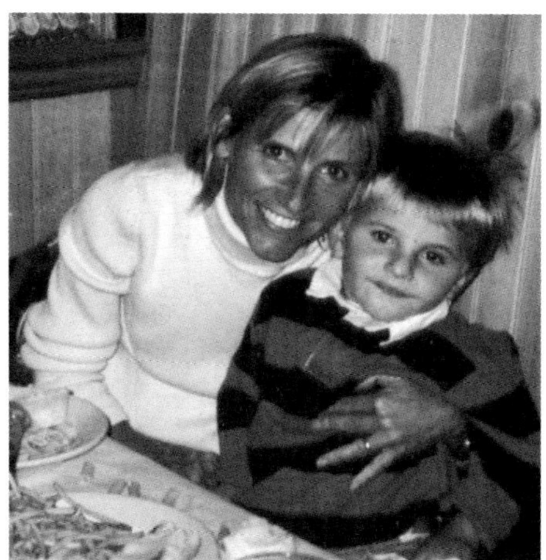

Benjamin was diagnosed at 2½ years

Biggest Challenge(s)

Every step we take, whether it be the diagnosis phase, scheduling and going to doctor's appointments (developmental pediatricians, opthamologist, audiologist, neurologist, GI specialist, nutritionists, etc.), researching on the internet (unending), making ready for blood, urine or stool tests and taking the tests, starting a new treatment or supplement, going on the GF/CF diet, waiting to see if a treatment is effective (including diet), backing off a treatment that produces side effects, etc. All these things take so much time. As they all add up, the clock is ticking and Benjamin is getting older. We're afraid we're losing the optimal developmental window that we read about. While he has made progress, he is not there yet and we are not clear if all these things will work. He doesn't talk well or understand things. Two years after we first suspected autism, Benjamin is now 4 1/2. Others tell us we are lucky to have had an early diagnosis, and with that we hoped (maybe naively) that he would be mainstreamed by kindergarten. Although he is 6 months away from age 5, we are feeling that he may not get there by then.

> "Most of the important things in the world have been accomplished by people who have kept on trying when there seemed to be no hope at all."
> – Dale Carnegie

Greatest Blessings

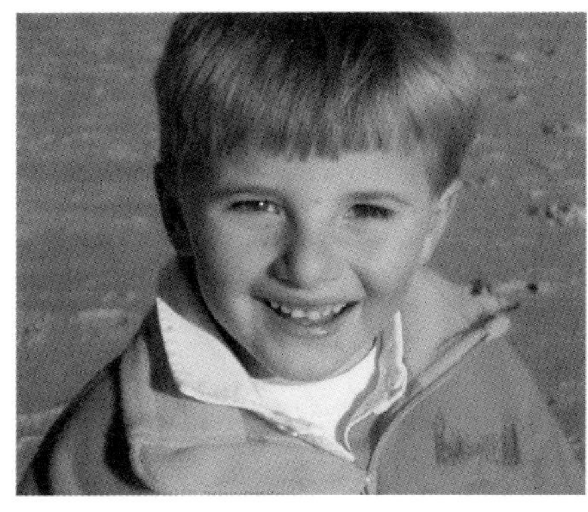

First blessing: Benjamin's school in Delaware. We moved to Delaware in 2000 for job-related reasons. We did not know Benjamin would be later diagnosed with autism and we would be needing autism services. Two years later we learned that we had, in fact, moved to a town with the largest public-school program for students with autism in the United States. Established more than 20 years ago, the Delaware Autism Program (DAP) is a nationally recognized autism program, awarded "Program of the Year" by the Autism Society of America in 2002. It seemed ironic that we were here, but truly a blessing. The specialists and teachers that work with Benjamin every day, year round, full-time are a blessing to Benjamin and have helped him so much to this point. This unique school with incredible services has the most caring staff of professionals we could hope for.

Other blessings: Benjamin. Benjamin is so beautiful, we sometimes can't believe there is anything wrong with him. My husband often says to me, "we make great kids" not even blinking an eye about Benjamin's autism because he is such a happy, energetic, beautiful boy and so is his loving big brother, Michael. We love our Benjamin and we know Benjamin loves us and he is a blessing to us no matter what.

Other blessings: Kind people. We have met so many people who have similar issues or other challenges in their families (usually more challenging than what we are dealing with). People seem to open up to you when you have an issue in your life and they share with you. They may have never opened up if they didn't know your situation. We have learned that almost everyone has issues and you get to know people better when you talk about them. We empathize better with people and we have become more generous with our time and money for the cause of autism and other causes because we see the importance of it.

Words of Wisdom

Take the time to do research and read about autism. Do this especially if you cannot afford specialists to guide you and do it even if you do have specialists. Research and read as much as you can so you can make informed decisions on what steps to take with your child and what questions to ask the professionals. There are tons of books on autism and the internet has a wealth of information available at no cost (except the time that it takes to go through it).

It is so easy to let life get in the way and just get by, or even give up without working to find a better life for your child. There are treatments and education services out there for your child. Autism just seems to be so complex that the answers are not clear cut. Don't let the clock tick away without making an effort and don't give up hope. We try to stay positive. We will not give up hope for Benjamin.

Tracy & Will

Tennessee

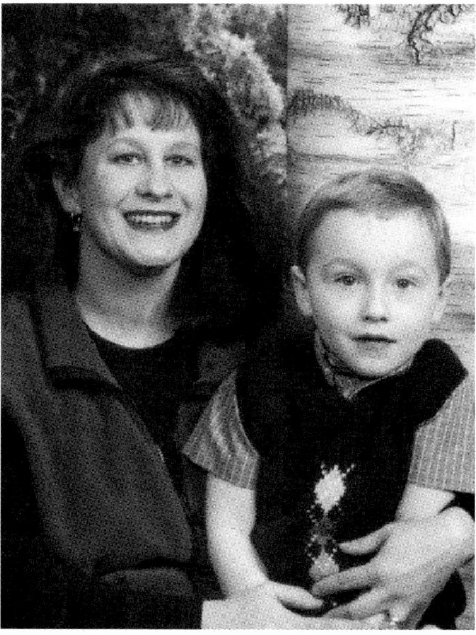

Will was diagnosed at 4 years

Contact:
thegotts@charter.net
NE Tennessee Autism Society Contact

Biggest Challenge(s)

Raising a child with autism is constantly a challenge! With society constantly bombarding us with the idealogy that perfection is the key to success in this world, our children just don't fit that notion and most never will.

I remember when I was pregnant with my son, I thought there wouldn't be anything I couldn't do for my child. I had such incredible plans! I had been a teacher in the public school system for the past six years. I would know how to raise a child who would love to learn! I didn't count on autism.

When my son was around the age of two and a half, the word autism was first mentioned to me by my son's speech and language therapist. I wanted to crawl into a deep dark hole. And for a while I actually did! I thought if I kept my son hidden from the world no one would realize he wasn't communicating. No one could hurt my son or I, if we just stayed hidden from the world. However, eventually, reality sets in and then comes that dreaded feeling, anger! Anger when no one seems to understand what you are going through.

Breaking loose from my hand and running from me in a public place happens to be one of my son's challenging behaviors. During a visit to our local hospital for some blood work, my son decided to pull his "escape act" by breaking loose from me while I was filling out an endless supply of paperwork. I proceeded to run right after my child as he zoomed down the hospital corridor passing numerous by-standers. I kept thinking to myself, "if only someone would just take the initiative to just stop him!" When all at once an elderly gentleman shouted at me, "Do you want to borrow my belt?" I wanted to shout obscenities at this man. How dare he! That day continues to haunt me because no one would reach out and simply help me. Our children are so normal looking that their disability doesn't stick out like a sore thumb.

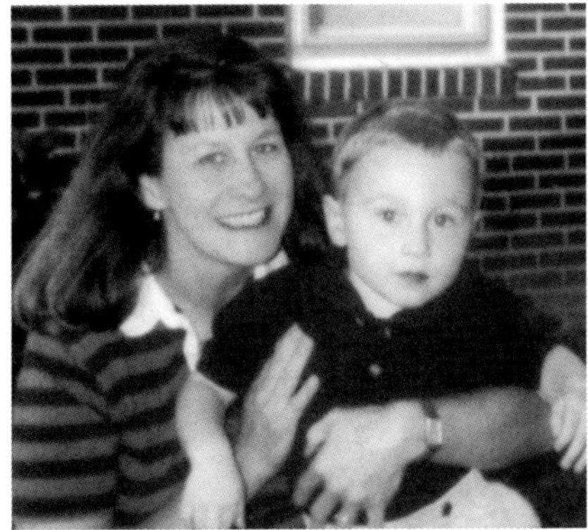

This is why I feel that autism awareness is the most important mission in my life. I owe it to my child and others like him, to bring this disability into the main stream of our society. Everyone needs to understand why our children act and communicate the way that they do.

Greatest Blessings

My greatest blessing is by far the everlasting expressions of love I receive everyday from my son. He lovingly gives me what I call "backward hugs." He presses his lips to my arm in an effort to kiss me! He is a dedicated mama's boy! He is part of my heart and soul.

The innocence of children is beautiful! I am a kindergarten teacher who experiences everyday the wisdom of a five year old. My son is mainstreamed with a full-time aide into the kindergarten room right next door. I am blessed for my child to have such a dedicated teacher who explains to her class that my son is the way that he is because of his autism and not because he does not want to be their friend.

My son's aide, "Mrs. B", is a blessing beyond words. Not only does she tirelessly never give up on my child, she never lets him give up on himself. She concentrates on what he can do and not what he can't do! Most importantly, she prays for him every day. What more can I ask for?!

Everyday I have the opportunity to observe first-hand the kindness of the children from the three kindergarten classes that my child is mixed with. I might see a child extending their hand to my son or offering a listening ear to words that I know they do not understand. It's a blessed experience that is simply hard to put into words.

Words of Wisdom

I remember feeling helpless after trying different diets and vitamin therapies to "cure" my child of his autism. When I continued to be discouraged, the director over my son's speech and language therapy program at our local state university, reminded me that the real "cure" for autism was in all the hard work. In other words, the "cure" is in the therapies. Speech and language, occupational, and physical therapies are the keys to success for our children! Once I realized this, my guilt subsided and I was able to get up every morning of every day and go to work for my son!

Tutta & Inka

Finland

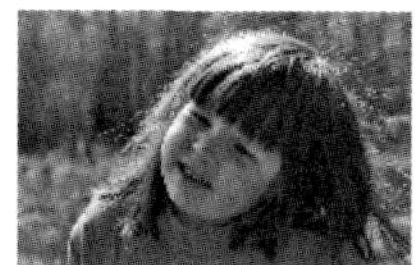

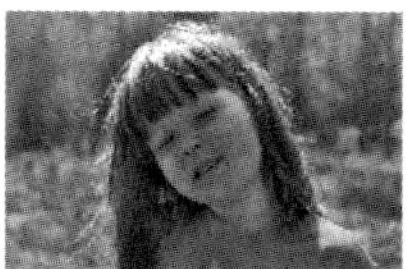

CONTACT:
tutta2@luukku.com
+358405152966

Inka was diagnosed at 4 years

BIGGEST CHALLENGE(S)

Inka-Annina is a 5-year-old girl with autism. Inka was at the age of 1 year and a half when I noticed that everything is not alright. But the diagnosis we got at the age of four.

There are a few main challenges which the parents of a child with autism could have. In Finland the parents have to fight really hard for the rights and appropriate services. You have to have the strength to do it. I myself felt it so wrong. It's really hard to have a child with autism and it should be enough. In the middle of processing that your child has autism, you have to fight with the people who should help your family and your child. You have to find yourself the information about the services for your child. Even though you are tired (because your child with autism will be sometimes hard to handle), remember that the early years are really important. Be honest to yourself, if you are tired, get help. Get as much information as you can about autism, but remember that your child is an individual.

The second big challenge is that people don't know much about autism. Even your relatives or friends don't automatically get information about it. You have to encourage them to communicate with your child, and tell them again and again how to treat your child. Don't get angry if people that you don't know will tell you how your child doesn't know how to behave or how you are a bad mother because your child cries at the shop, etc. They just don't understand what autism is.

At first it would be hard when you notice that your family's social life will die. You can't participate in every party or happening because your child can't bear them. But little by little your child bears more. Get a good nanny for your child sometimes and go out with the rest of the family.

If you have in your family other children, it will be a great challenge to have a normal family life. Try to have it.

Greatest Blessings

Although it's hard with the child with autism, there are also the moments of great blessings. The first eye-contact you will remember forever. The laughing together is something you can't describe. When you really are in contact with the child, it's so total. When your child laughs, it will come right from her heart. When your child is happy, you sure are too.

I myself have few persons to whom I will be grateful for the rest of my life. Thank you to my dear husband for listening to my sorrows in nights and days, to understanding my deep sorrow in bad times and the great moments with Inka in good times. Thank you to my parents for helping me with the other children, and when I was very tired you took care of Inka. Thank you to my friend Marjo for listening to me and my sorrows. Thank you to Felix and Lisel and the whole Tuomaskallio-koti for taking so good care of Inka. Thank you to my brother Aki for treating Inka as any other of my children.

Words of Wisdom

The words of wisdom to friends and relatives: help the family. You can get the other children and go with them for example, to cinema, to skating, anything. Get the parents a free evening sometimes; go to their home and take care of the children so that the parents can do something together. Understand that the family is sometimes very tired. Listen to them and their sorrows. You notice soon who are the real friends, and they are a great blessing to you.

> "The first eye-contact you will remember forever. The laughing together is something you can't describe. When you really are in contact with the child, it's so total."

Val & Shelly

Texas

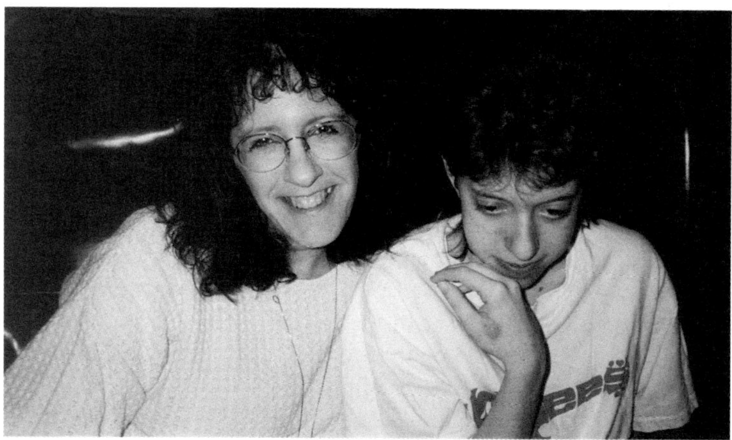

Shelly at 20 years old

Shelly was diagnosed at 36 months

CONTACT:

val@companyidentities.com

BIGGEST CHALLENGE(S)

The first challenge was going through the steps of mourning, because the child I gave birth to wasn't the same child that sat on the other side of the two-way mirror. The experts gathered to assess my first born. Then almost 3, Shelly had bewildered some of them, but endeared herself to them all. So many questions had come with me that day. Why doesn't Shelly speak? Why did it take so long for her to stand and walk? Will she ever catch up with her peers? The white coated doctor at the head of the conference table stood, ready to speak for all the other white coats. I braced myself for the worst. The new life inside me, baby number two, squirmed as I reached for the tissue box in the middle of the table. I wondered how many other parents had sat here before me, crying?

"Shelly's hearing is intact," said the examining physician. "Vision, intact. But according to the Gesell Developmental Assessment, she is well below normal in fine and gross motor." His words were bits of crushed ice tumbling down my spine. Who's this Gesell guy? "Shelly's gait is wide-based and immature for her age. Her arms are frequently at mid-guard." After three days of testing, tell me something I don't already know. "She has postural and tactile defensiveness. She'll never run. Never ride a bike. Probably never read, write, or speak like her peers," he said. His peers nodded in agreement.

First stage of grief... anger. Who the hell did this "expert" think he was, painting such a bleak picture of Shelly's future? How could he know these negative things after spending only 15 minutes with her over the last three days?

"What the hell is wrong with my daughter!" I blurted out. A heavy silence answered back. All the white coats turned towards me. I didn't care. I came to this famous clinic in Houston's world renowned Medical Center to get answers, damn it! "It is our finding that Shelly is autistic, mentally retarded and has fine and gross motor and speech delays."

My hands protectively touched my belly. Was the child inside of me destined for the same diagnosis? Did some genetic monster invade our family tree? White Coat droned on but I'd heard enough. When he was through, he asked me if I had any questions. I looked at Shelly on the other side of a two-way mirror as she rocked her body and tapped on her chin. 'No questions', was all I could say. I gathered up all of Shelly's have-to-have toys and put them in the diaper bag. Shelly looked happy to be leaving. At the car, I buckled her in her car seat and placed a folder full of reports next to her on the back seat. As I drove home, the windows were down and Shelly's baby fine hair was blowing wild and free. Her breathing became rapid, as it always did on car rides. My heart cracked. Depression... the next stage of grief.

"It doesn't matter what they say, Shelly." I gripped the steering wheel tighter, trying to hide my pain. "If you want to run, you'll run. If you want to ride a bike, by God, you'll ride a bike. You may be autistic but you're still a Mark, and we're a stubborn lot." Denial... another stage of grief.

Eight-year old Shelly has challenged me at shoe stores. She doesn't like her feet touched at all. She screams a lot, every day, and I can usually take it in stride after so many years. But when we go out in public, I can't help thinking people are judging me as a parent. If they only knew.

Shelly is afraid of everything. Her shoulders tense whenever she walks down the hall. She's afraid of noises, so I vacuum the house when she's at school. And trains! Forget about it! She's very tactilely defensive, especially around her neck, head and feet. I never bring her with me to buy shoes anymore. I buy them, bring them home and deal with her there.

A solution. That's a challenge. Finding solutions to all the differences our family endures. Shelly has to have things pretty much the same every day. Robyn, her sister, born neurologically-typical, thank you God, and I try to accommodate her. Robyn appointed herself Shelly's other parent as soon as she understood that her sister was not like other people. I struggled with guilt about that, but I needed her. Their father was gone.

It is such a challenge dealing with it all. I smile and act noble, but inside I'm full of guilt and resentment. I can't believe I'm still bathing her! Soon she'll have breasts. Will she tolerate a bra? And then there's her period. All young women get their period, no matter what their mental capacity.

The challenge of communication was enormous. At eight years old, Shelly started to say things, although mostly gibberish. To communicate, I used every means possible. Sign language, the written word, body language and speech. Shelly learned what words go with what situations. She'd say "eat," I fed her. She'd say "juice," I gave her juice. I waited an eternity for her to say "mommy". Now, she says "mommy"over and over again. I know she wants to say more, but she can't. In frustration, she bites her hand. There's a large, hard callous there now. There were days that I hated it. Shelly hated it more I think. But when Shelly makes eye contact with me, it's a gift from God.

Greatest Blessings

Family is the biggest blessing. My parents live close by and are always there to help in every way. When Shelly turned 18, her peers graduated from high school. Shelly remained behind, though, for a few more years of special education. Robyn attended the same school. Robyn's tolerance and patience still amazes me. She's never embarrassed to point Shelly out to her friends. If they ever use the word "retarded", she tells them not to say that about someone.

I elected to stop Shelly's periods. It was just too much for her, for her caregivers at school and for me. I struggled for years with that decision. Now it's a blessing. I've met so many supportive people over the course of Shelly's life. Some had children much worse off than Shelly. Some had children that were less challenged. I've often wished Shelly were less handicapped. At least we'd be communicating.

The rapid breathing she did on car rides became full-blown seizures, and she's had as many as 25 a day for years. Recently, we found Topamax and Gabitril, two anti-seizure medications, and her seizures decreased. Then, Shelly's neurologist told us about the Vegas Nerve Stimulator, an implanted device that attaches to the Vegas nerve in the neck and sends an electrical impulse to the brain every 3 minutes for 30 seconds. Shelly underwent the implantation better than anyone expected. No more seizures and Shelly's speech and eye contact improved, too. A medical blessing. Two ABA therapists come to our house and work with her in all areas and we all see improvement. These two women are so well trained. I thank God for what they've taught, not only Shelly, but Robyn and me as well.

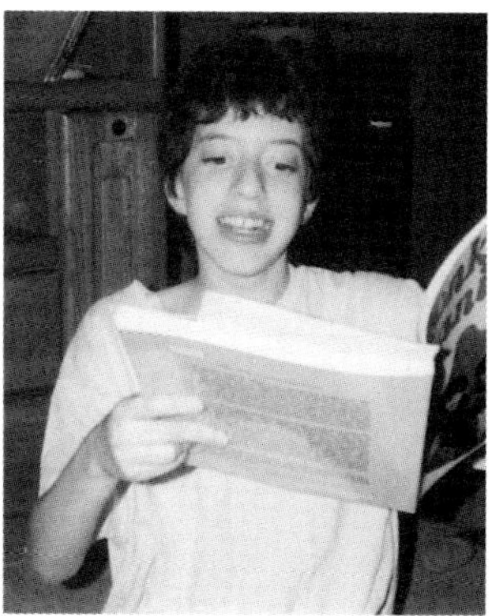

Words of Wisdom

Don't ever give up on finding everything that could possibly help your child be all he/she can be. No one will ever come knocking on your door to help you. You have to get out there and explore all the possibilities.

Shelly is now 22 and out of school. She's still living with Robyn and me. I found one of Shelly's therapist through MHMR and the other through the Houston school district. I also found grants to help pay for them. There are more resources available now then when Shelly was first diagnosed.

Have patience but separate yourself from your child if frustration takes over. Do what you can, but get help for what you can't do. I believe it was Hillary Clinton that said, "It takes a village to raise a child." Raising a child with autism takes a team of educated, caring professionals, doctors aware of what's new in treatment and research, and a loving family.

We're three women living special lives together now, Shelly, Robyn and I. Shelly's the most interesting person I know, and I'm very proud to be 'Shelly's Mommy.'

And guess what Dr. White Coat… Shelly was a Bat Mizvah at age 12. She reads, can bathe herself, stuff envelopes and sort objects. She can dress herself with little assistance and sometimes speaks spontaneously. She can operate the VCR and CD player and loves Crayola® crayons, rock and roll music, and shopping on eBay.

Verla & Clint

Kansas

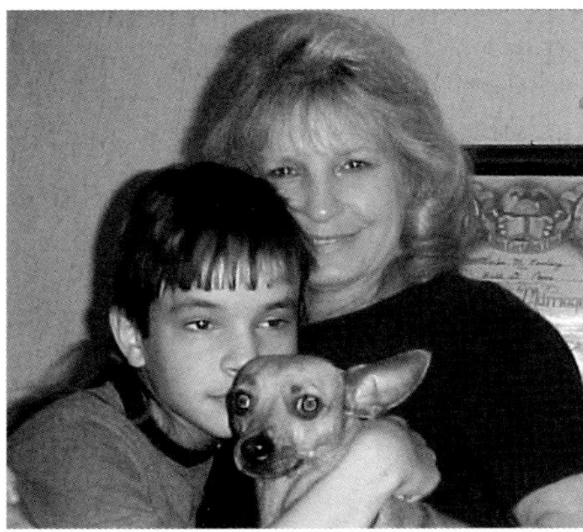

Clint at 13
Jake & Mom

CONTACT:
verlap@wheatstate.com

Clint was diagnosed at 2½ years

BIGGEST CHALLENGE(S)

The biggest challenges in having a child with special needs, such as autism, are a combination of many. To try and find balance in life would be one of mine. After you get a diagnosis of autism you take on many occupations. You try to juggle and learn many different jobs and thus you become:

An Educator – Learning all about autism and finding ways to reach and work with your child. You help educate those who are not familiar with autism, even your child's doctors and teachers, to help aide in the urgency of early intervention – which is key with a child with autism.

A Lawyer – You learn the law so you know your child's rights in his school settings, in the community, and in the everyday life. Educate yourself regarding your child's insurance plan and be prepared to appeal a hearing.

A Therapist – You have to learn about occupational therapy and adaptive physical therapy. You learn about sensory integration in order to help calm your child and help him overcome fears of things like loud sounds, too much noise distraction, new environments, smells, and eye contact. You learn to be a speech therapist so you can help your child communicate at home, school and with family and friends. You try to help them become independent and communicate their wants and needs.

A Doctor – You learn to determine if your child is sick when the communication isn't there for him to express that he is sick or where it is that he is hurting. You learn to read the signs and symptoms of anything from a toothache, to a sore throat, or ear

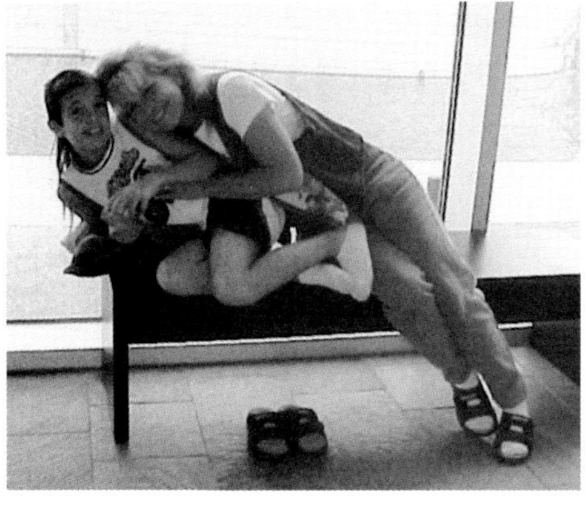

infection. You learn what behaviors indicate that your child may be sick or hurting.

You juggle all these jobs in addition to trying to remain a good wife – being able to give your husband attention or even the TIME that there never seems to be enough of. And then there is the most important role for me, the one of the loving Mother. That is the number ONE importance with my child. I also have to give time to my daughter, to let her know that I love both children the same, although sometimes more time and attention is given to Clint.

I have learned that trying to balance all of these "jobs" does not happen on an even keel. You do the very best you can. You learn to accept that all things cannot get done in a day and know that you have to take the time for yourself to help balance a "mom's day."

Greatest Blessings

Having a child with autism has shown me that I have many blessings that I don't think I would have been able to see in my life if not for Clint. One of the blessings is that I have learned how very hard it is for Clint, who is now thirteen, to struggle almost every single day of his life to try to accept things in his world that are not easy for him. He has overcome so many things by the hard and dedicated work that he has done. Working with Clint, I have realized that I have taken for granted how "easy" it is to learn something new. With Clint you must break down each task one small step at a time until you reach the full concept of what you are teaching him.

I am blessed to have a daughter who is an amazing sister to Clint – a sister who has always loved and cared for her brother unconditionally. She is fifteen years old, and twenty two months older than Clint. Clint did not even recognize her as an object, or person, until one day at the age of four when he started looking at her and wanting her participation and help in his daily life. It was an amazing day for all of us! He just started looking into her eyes and smiling. He had always noticed her, but never let it be known until that day.

To have a husband who is a loving father and commits himself to being a dad that is going to be by his children's side all of their life is a gift. To be faced with the challenges, and the reality of how hard life can be, turns around for me if I notice that Clint, being who he is, is a gift. The humor he provides shows us that we should not to take life so serious in this ever fast and stressing world.

I am one of the very fortunate parents who have been blessed with wonderful and caring teachers in my child's life since his diagnosis. As a parent you should be treated as an equal member of your son's educational team. By educating myself, to the best of my ability, I have been able to be knowledgeable enough coming to the IEP meetings to be a productive part in his educating process. I have always been treated fairly and with respect as part of the IEP team. The special educator in charge of my son's academic process has been a blessing – like an angel sent from heaven. She has gone beyond what her professional title indicates, and I believe you have to have that type of person to have a successful education program. To know when to push, and when you are about to push too much, is a special skill. Clint has been blessed with great paraprofessionals. They have been consistent through years and thus we have not had to overcome the challenges that come with someone new being introduced into his life. The love and support of my parents and sisters are another blessing Clint and I have in our lives.

Words of Wisdom

The words of wisdom that I would pass on to others would be:

- Read Temple Grandin's book, *Thinking in Pictures*. It helped me to find out what was going on in Clint's mind – the mind of a person with autism was a world I knew nothing about before my son's diagnosis.
- Get positive support. Definitely connect with other parents of children with autism. Find a support group, whether it be on the internet or through groups that are active somewhere close to where you live.
- Take time-outs for yourself.
- Give your child times to be who he is so that he may adapt to our world. Allow their personalities to become part of the family. Each member of your family has a personality and you will be rewarded by allowing their gift of giving of themselves.
- Stay one step ahead, always. Accept that you always do your best, even when you doubt yourself and the "only if" phrases come into your head.

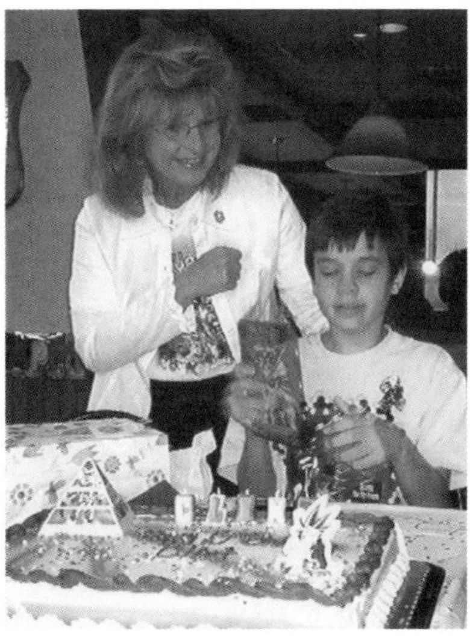

Vicki & Sam

Kansas

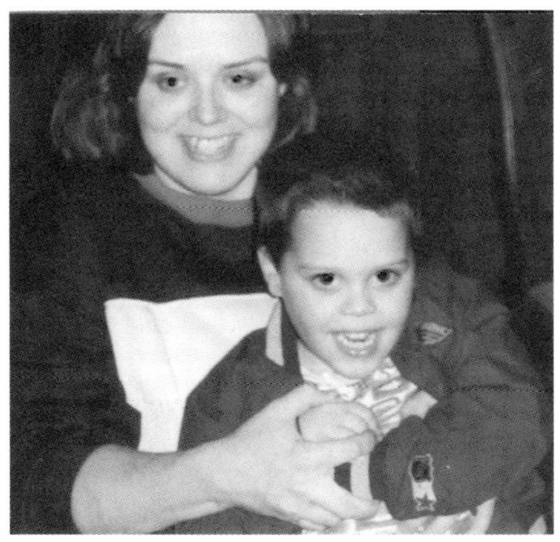

Sam 3 years old

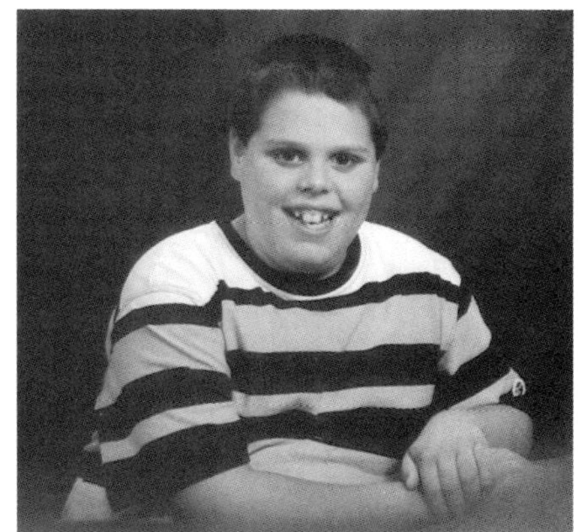

Sam 12 years old

Sam was diagnosed at 2 years

Biggest Challenge(s)

My name is Vicki and I am the mother of three beautiful kids, two girls, ages 15 and 11, and a 14-year-old boy named Sam, who has autism. We just moved last year to Kansas from O'Fallon, Missouri where we lived for the previous 11 years.

Sam likes pizza and French fries, Disney movies, books, and computer and video games. He's always been REALLY into animals, and currently dinosaurs. He is verbal, though not a big conversationalist, and at times it is difficult for him to make people understand what he is trying to say.

One of the biggest challenges for me was overcoming how his diagnosis of autism changed my perception of my son. It was like they had taken away my beautiful, perfect little boy, whose future was so full of possibilities, and returned to me a fragile little stranger who had a label that I knew nothing about, except that there was no cure. I was afraid that if I did something wrong, I'd make things worse. So, for the next several years, I second-guessed my every decision regarding Sam. How should I respond to his behaviors? How do we discipline him without reinforcing negative behaviors? Should we try medication or behavioral therapy? The list goes on and on. Finally, when Sam was in first grade, I figured out that, even if I made a mistake, Sam would be okay. Parents make mistakes all the time, that's how we learn to be better parents.

Other challenges include:
• Sam's tendency towards aggression when he is mad or frustrated, or sometimes when he is over-stimulated.
• Decisions regarding therapies and medications – when to start, which ones to try, and changing them when necessary.
• Getting our former school district to accommodate Sam's needs – teachers rarely have enough functional knowledge of autism and school districts are reluctant to provide more than minimal training, as it is expensive.
• Since moving to a new town, it's been difficult finding new supports, especially respite, and you get moved to the bottom of a new waiting list for funding aids.

Greatest Blessings

Sometimes we can get bogged down by all the problems we face but there are blessings if you look for them. Hearing Sam say a new phrase or watching him master a new task, little things that you'd normally take for granted, are so special. When he hugs me or tells me he loves me, it's like no other feeling in the world.

When I close my eyes and try to picture Sam differently, I can't. I love him as he is. While there are many things that I'm sorry he probably will never do, I'm glad that he is less likely to become addicted to drugs or alcohol. It's unlikely that he will ever bring home a girlfriend that I don't approve of. And I selfishly find comfort in that I'll never have to send my son off to war.

Other blessings:
• Seeing Sam's sisters go out of their way to help when he is having a rough time makes me realize how Sam is helping them to learn about compassion for others.
• Some of the very dedicated therapists, teachers and paraprofessionals Sam's been fortunate to have – I hope you know how special you are.
• Our respite providers – you guys are terrific!
• The Judevine Center for Autism in St. Louis County – I can't say thank you enough. You guys and gals are the best, bar-none! Thanks, Mrs. B.!

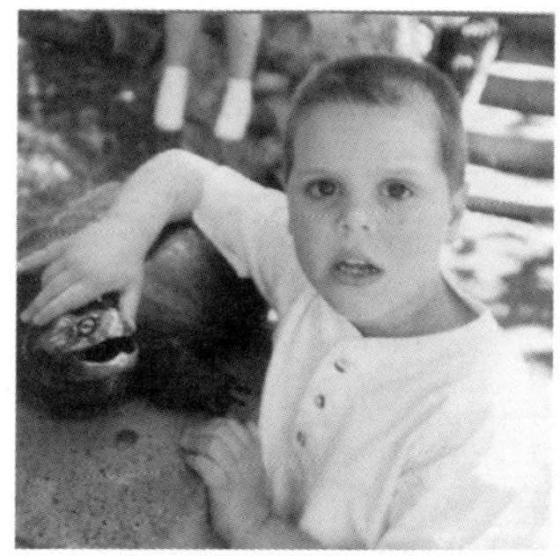

Words of Wisdom

Don't be afraid to reach out. Even if you're not the support group type, go to one occasionally. You'll meet contacts, find out information about services, providers, and resources. And sometimes, you just need to talk (yell, scream, cry – insert your word of choice) to someone who knows exactly what you're dealing with. I can talk to my sister, who I know cares and loves me, and she never fails to say the wrong thing to me. I can meet someone at a support meeting; know nothing about them except that they have a child on the spectrum, and talk, meaningfully, for an hour or two. And sometimes come away with (or share) valuable new insights or information.

Don't go to IEP meetings alone – always bring an advocate or at least a friend for support!

Vicky & Elizabeth

Illinois

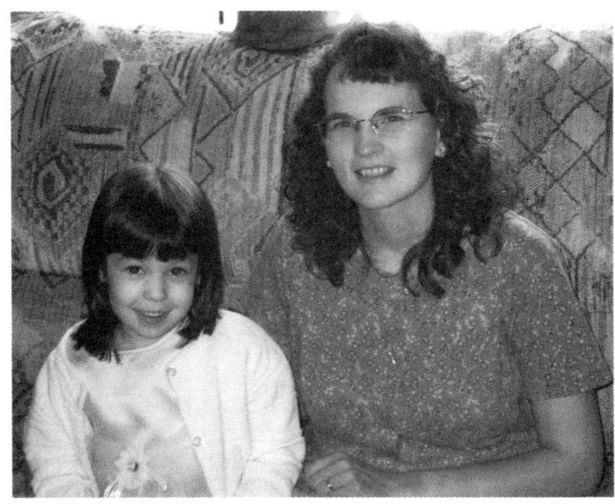

Contact:
davick92@yahoo.com

Elizabeth was diagnosed at 2½ years

Biggest Challenge(s)

When my daughter, Elizabeth, was diagnosed with autism at the age of 2½, my husband and I began the most challenging journey we have ever faced. We encountered difficult decisions, such as which treatments and therapies would be best for Elizabeth, how to manage the cost of each intervention, who to go to for professional help, behavioral issues, potty training delays, communication dilemmas, and many other challenges. We tried several interventions, including (but not limited to) Speech/Occupational/Physical therapies, special diets, secretin injection, chelation therapy, digestive enzymes, Ambrotose Complex, and other dietary supplements. Each thing we've tried has been a challenge in and of itself. Then, on top of everything, the biggest challenge has been the testing of our faith. Before Elizabeth came along, my husband and I had gone through some difficulties with infertility, so we knew our newborn daughter was truly a gift from God. Because of this, I personally went through a very difficult time of grieving for the normalcy of my child.

As a mother, I had so many hopes and plans for my child. I wanted her to excel as a student and as a person, one day fall in love, get married, and have children of her own. Why wouldn't God want this for my daughter as well? I experienced shock, numbness, hurt, fear, sorrow, and anger, all at different times. But, I've learned that, with testing, comes strength; and, with strength, the ability to cope in difficult situations. Through this experience, I am stronger in my faith and believe God truly does know what is best for me. I don't believe He caused Elizabeth's autism, but He did allow it to happen for a reason. So, instead of being bitter and angry, I have chosen to make the best of my situation, and use it to bring hope and encouragement to others.

Greatest Blessings

Elizabeth has made wonderful progress over the years and has overcome many obstacles. She continues to improve and we feel so blessed to have her in our lives. One particularly blessed event was when Elizabeth called me "mommy" for the first time. It is always very special when a mother hears her child call her "mommy" but, with Elizabeth, I had to wait 4½ years before she actually made the connection to who I was. It was music to my ears!

Words of Wisdom

Being a Christian does not mean everything will be perfect in my life. But, I have allowed God to help me make it through the difficult times. I know I can always rely on Him to give me the wisdom and strength I need. (James 1:5, Psalm 28:7)

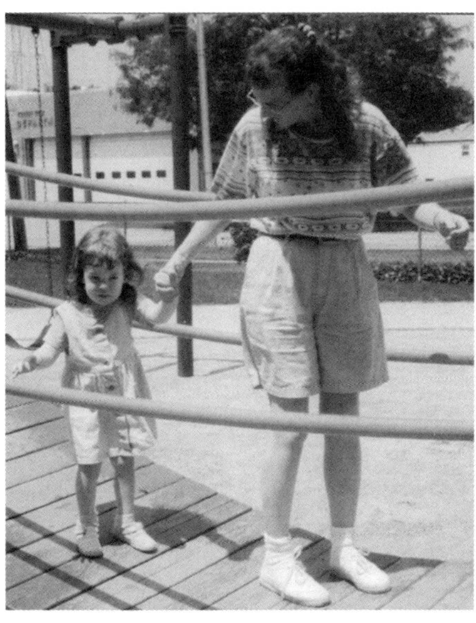

Virginia, David & Aaron

Florida

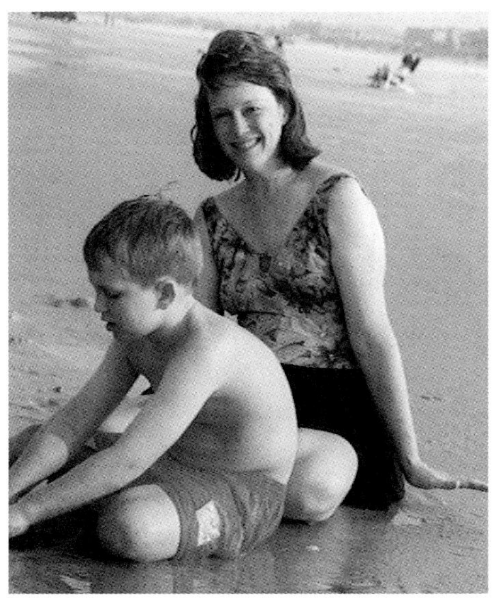

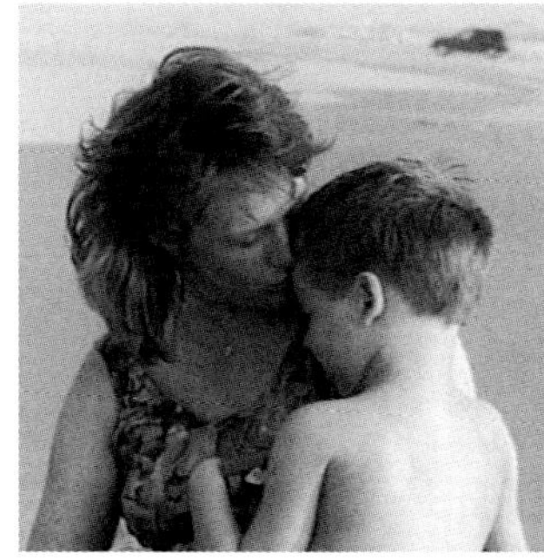

David was diagnosed at 2½ years
Aaron was diagnosed at 18 months

CONTACT:
mccormacboys@peoplepc.com

BIGGEST CHALLENGE(S)

We are a family caught in the intricate sticky web of autism spun by an unseen hand – the patterns shift, two steps back, one step forward. I remain in the center empowered by a love so deep that I am staggered over and over. I celebrate, I weep, I pray and I pray – I pray to understand, to encourage, to discover, for patience and then with a fresh breath of confidence I release – I release the fear, the uncertainties, the medical issues, the bizarre behaviors, the melt downs, the violence, the educational woes – and I begin again – a new day colored as bright as the rainbows that pour from David's soul; a day filled with activities as ceaseless as Aaron's jabbering.

Greatest Blessings

We all make our way bound by that common thread of love that weaves our family's days; I've seen God give my husband such amazing strength and grace in the midst of an autistic storm that rips through our home like a tornado. By HIS sustaining power I manage to maintain like one of those weighted punch toys that pops back up after you knock it down. The boys live their moments in unique simplicity – unfettered with typical concerns yet bound within this mysterious web. Their ability to adapt is amazing.

There are moments I call 'heart takes flight' – like:

- The sound of David's lyrical "Mommy, where are you?" still takes my breath away.
- Aaron singing, "When Your Heart is Full of Love" by Fred Rogers. I had just returned from a weekend autism conference and he just launched into the complete song, all the verses, melody – I sat there amazed.
- David telling a little boy at the YMCA pool his name – only we special parents know this joy.
- Aaron's adorable yoga variations – like 'tired pose'.
- David singing "You are the Lamb of God" holding the baby Jesus figurine from the manger scene, or reciting Mr. Roger's affirmation that there is no one exactly like you and people can like you just as you are.

Words of Wisdom

We witness miracles in simple ways – in this we can actually thank God for our thorn in the flesh. Psalm 90:9 says, "We live our lives as a tale that is told", another translation reads "as a web that is spun". The reality of autism is with me as I go to sleep and in the morning as I open my eyes – and even in my dream states. The "why" nags at my mind almost constantly but the joy, strength, energy, creativity and innocence that I witness in my sons take me to new heights – and I yield into God's perfect plan and purpose in our lives.

"The boys live their moments in unique simplicity – unfettered with typical concerns yet bound within this mysterious web. Their ability to adapt is amazing."

Marge & Jennifer

by Judy

The most important blessing for Jill is the two women who opened up their hearts and their homes to help me care for her when we had no one.

My mother was dying in 1994, I was divorced, and Jill had been struggling in the school system for years. Emotionally, physically, and financially there wasn't much left of me. After moving her from one school to the next and finally to another lower-functioning school; Jill had had enough. She came home from her 'new school', frustrated at not being able to tell me that someone had dragged her across the floor, causing a rug-burn on her back; and physically attacked me for the first time. Not realizing her own strength, she grabbed my hair and yanked me to the ground. On my knees, I began to pray, It is then I learned the meaning of 'Let Go and Let God'. He was surely watching over us because He sent us Marge and her family.

Marge took Jill on an emergency respite situation and it was no mistake that the district she lived in was one in which they had a successful Autism (ABA) program. Jill was only supposed to be with Marge for 10 days to give me a rest. But then I met Kevin, the Autism Specialist, who told me he could help her if I enrolled her in the ABA program in Marge's district. I made the decision to allow her to stay with this family during the week. The hardest decision I ever had to make was admitting I could no longer raise her alone. The only thing I knew about this family was they were willing to take Jill <u>knowing she had autism</u> and that God had sent them to us. I had to trust His guidance.

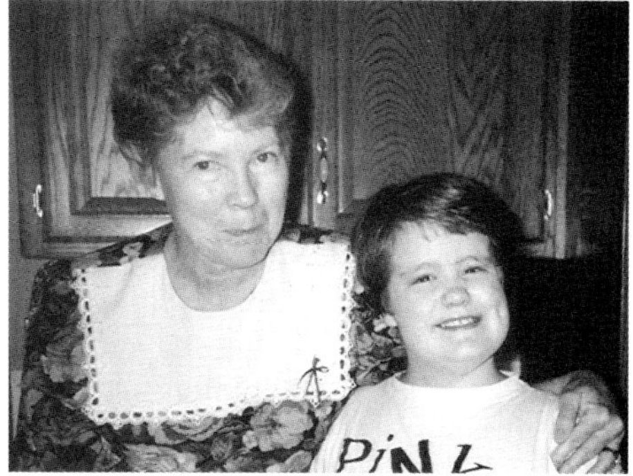

Marge & Jill, April 1994

Years later when Marge's husband died, Jill came back to live with me full-time. Things were going well until changes were made in that ABA program. Significant staff left and it basically fell apart. Jill suffered immensely. The stress and strain finally took its toll on me, my relationship, my other children, and I found myself, once again, asking for help.

My only saving grace was Jennifer. She was one of Jill's teachers from that once-successful autism program who left because she felt unsupported by school administrators. Still, she was the only 'autism expert' left in the area.

She was my <u>*only*</u> hope.

Jennifer turned Jill's life around. I continue to be amazed at how well Jill does with her guidance, I hardly recognize my own daughter talking in complete sentences, making herself something to eat, recognizing the dog is scratching at the door and she lets him in! Jill still requires 24/7 supervision but her progress is amazing! Jennifer has such supportive friends, family, and a church community that have all lovingly and unconditionally accepted Jill into their lives.

On Jill's 21st birthday, after she opened presents, the phone rang; much to my surprise it was for Jill. "Gram", Jennifer's mom, was calling to wish Jill a Happy Birthday. It was all I could do to keep from tearing up from seeing how much they truly cared about her. Not only has Jennifer and her family helped me with Jill but Jennifer's mom and dad help her too. I don't tell them often enough how this means the world to me, because I can no longer give Jill grandparents. My greatest fear has always been 'who will care for her when I am gone'. Right before my eyes are God's angels, Jennifer and Ryan and their two children, Madison and Remington; and Jennifer's parents, Gram and Papa, loving her and caring for her straight from their heart. I don't know where we'd be without them.

There is not enough money in the world to ever repay them all for what they have done for me and my daughter. I know they were heaven-sent. Not only am I forever grateful for all they have given, I love them dearly and know they are our most precious gifts from God.

I asked Jennifer to also contribute her heartfelt thoughts because she now knows what it is like to raise a child with autism. Here is what she shared:

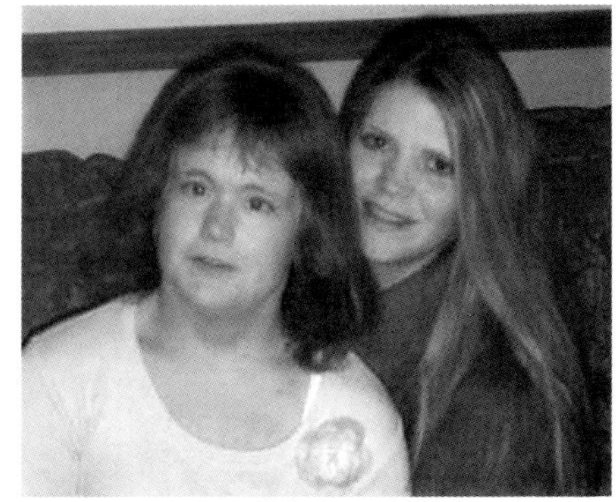
Jill & Jenn, 2005

Biggest Challenge(s)

The biggest challenges I have with Jill are not really with Jill. They are how others treat her. As soon as people notice something different about her they treat her differently. Our biggest challenge is in encouraging others to let Jill be the best she can be. She is such a smart, capable, loving person who needs to feel important.

Then there is a definite balancing act that is ongoing with my other two children. The other day our 11-year-old was distraught over a Latin test score. When I asked her why she didn't just tell me, she said, "I'm supposed to be the easy one."

Greatest Blessings

Achievements for Jill, like being put in front (in charge) of the production line after starting at the end (with constant supervision). Losing almost 100 pounds when food is such a huge reinforcer! Watching her make a pumpkin pie with my Mom and giving me a thumb's up and saying "Are you proud?" The excitement as she runs up the driveway from the school bus because she's happy to be home. Watching her sing praise and worship at church. Knowing that God has brought her to our lives *to better us*. Judy: She had the courage to let go and let Jill move on with our family, it was a huge leap of faith and we are eternally grateful.

Words of Wisdom

Expect the best. Keep the bar high so that the children are able to show you what they are capable of. Let them be important as well as productive. Know that this is just for now, when you meet in heaven they will be whole and able to thank you for the piggy back ride you gave them here on Earth.

In loving memory of
Ryan Long
1984 — 2003

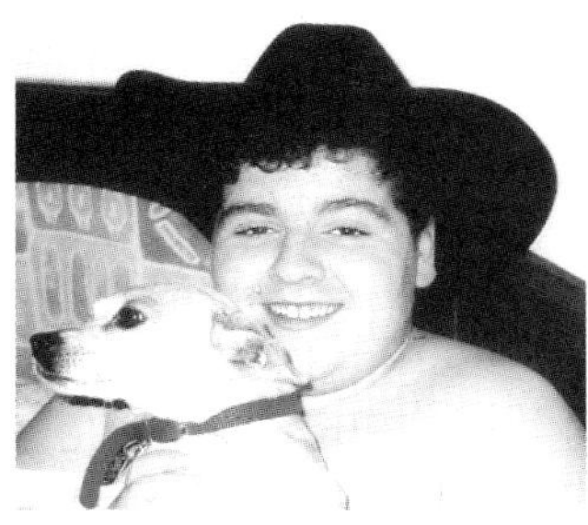

Ryan spent years in the Autism (ABA) program with Jill and also shared her exact birthday. We miss him dearly. To his mom, Diane — bless you for being the light in his life and for being one of 'us' — a mother of a child with autism, need I say more?! Jennifer E. so eloquently said to Diane when Ryan died, "you don't need to be his voice anymore because he will have his own voice."

I asked Diane to contribute something and she said that Ryan was her Blessing and then shared this letter she wrote to Ryan on his birthday, almost one year after his passing.

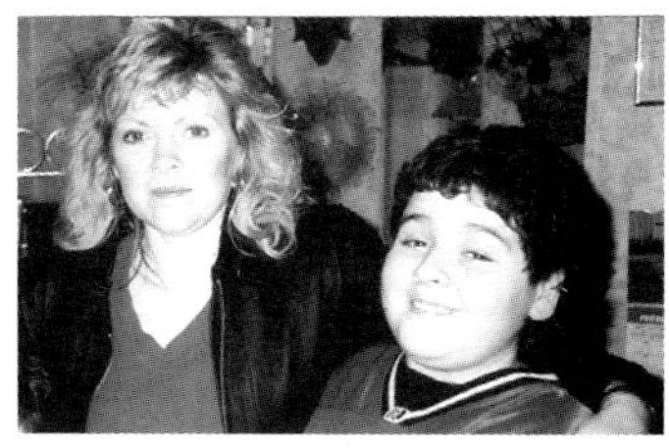

January 6, 2004

Dear Ryan,

Happy Birthday,
I love you and I miss you so very much.
I am hurting so bad. Are you okay? Please let me know if you are doing okay.
If you can please, let me know if you are okay.
January 6, 1984 the day you were born was the best day of my life, and August 11, 1988 when your brother Jeff was born was too.
I know you love me like I love you; I think I could be okay if I know you are okay.
I want to know that you are warm. I want to know that you are safe and happy.
I want to know that you are surrounded by loving souls who are helping you.
Maybe you do not need help anymore; maybe you can take care of yourself just fine.
I want to know all these things about you.
I am worried about you and I worry about how you are doing without me.
I miss you so much. My heart is broken, but how I do wish you are doing okay.
I want you to GO FOR IT TOO. Someday we will be together again.

Love, Mom

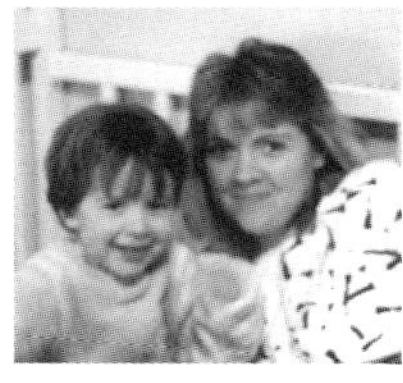

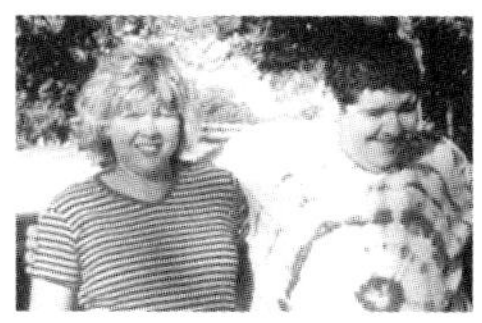

Diane also said that she was in her van and the windows were all fogged up. She remembered that Ryan loved writing on the fogged up windows and when she looked over at the window she saw where he must've written "Go for it' and she knew there was her sign that he is okay.

Mother's in Action

Some of the mothers who have submitted entries to this book have initiated, or are involved in, some special programs, activities, and/or organizations listed below in no specific order.

Kalma

Started the Hawaii Chapter of Cure Autism Now (CAN) Foundation in 2003
www.cureautismnow.com

Adrianne

A volunteer on the Special Needs Committee of the Illinois Christian Home Educators. She would be pleased to help any and all who may be considering homeschooling, so please feel free to contact her at jeffelbe@earthlink.net

Bobbie

Recently founded an Autism/Aspergers Family Support Group in Kansas and would like to service the families that reside in Butler, Chase, Coffey, Greenwood, Lyon, Morris and Osage counties. Contact AASFSG@sbcglobal.net for further information.

Laura

You can visit her website at www.laurasantos.com and click on "about laura" to read more about her and her son. There is also a video clip about autism.

Phyllis

Founded a support group in the area (Washington) for the GFCF diet called D.I.S.H. (Dietary Interventions, Support and Hope), and works as the New Parent Liaison for special education preschool. For the local autism society she is the Information Officer. She also works in conjunction with her support group as a consultant for the GFCF diet for parents and schools (she helps the teachers set up a GFCF environment and understand the needs of their GFCF student) She loves to help others! Contact information is 360-636-6018 or dzerman2@yahoo.com

Unlocking Autism

A phenomenal website for parents www.unlockingautism.org
There is a representative from each state that parents can contact.

Moms who are Unlocking Autism Representatives for their state:

Theresa ~ CT	April ~ AR	Marie ~ TX
Angie ~ OR	LeAnne ~ WI	Michelle ~ TX
Teresa - OK	Kara ~ IA	

Author's Note: I was so impressed with this, as I read through the website, it brought tears to my eyes and a renewed hope for my daughter's future to possibly have something similar for her in our area. Anyone wanting to make a donation toward making this dream a reality for Jill & other young women, please contact me at Judy@AutismThoughts.com (or AutismThoughts@yahoo.com).

Ruthie

Mandy's Farm

www.MandysFarm.org - A new Ray of Hope

(taken directly from their webpage)

As parents or guardians of a young woman with autism, age 18 to 30, the time is nearing for you to do what you lovingly must - and plan for her future, as she transitions from home or school to another place and life.

But there are difficult, soul-searching questions. Where will she find the same loving care that you embraced and protected her with? Who can you trust to lead your child, as you would want, for the rest of her life? And yes, what will happen to her when you're no longer here? For these important reasons, for your precious daughter, Mandy's Special Farm exists.

Located on the outskirts of Albuquerque, New Mexico, Mandy's Special Farm - with more than four picturesque acres for living, learning, working and playing - is a shining, new ray of hope for young women with autism who likely will never live independently, as well as those who love them.

The mission of Mandy's Special Farm is to provide highest quality, long term, 24-hour care for a maximum six women with autism, ages 18 to 30 on admission.

The goal is to help these women achieve their greatest self-sufficiency, within a caring, structured, positive, purposeful, encouraging home-like atmosphere. And the hope? That six young women with autism will lead a better life - and that the parents of these special children will find peace of heart and mind.

Michelle

MichelleMGuppy@yahoo.com

www.TexasAutismAdvocacy.org (281) 686-0103

List owner and facilitator of Texas-Autism-Advocacy@yahoogroups.com, and corresponding website of resources & information, www.TexasAutismAdvocacy.org

Also, a Regional Coordinator for Partners Resource Network in Texas, which is a non-profit organization whose goal is to help parents to be effective, equal partners with professionals in the growth and education of their children. Partners Resource Network offers training, information, and support to parents of children with all types of disabilities. Website: www.PartnersTX.org

Christine H.

Autism Advocates of Indiana, Inc.

Co-Founder, Co-President www.AAIwalk.org

Partners in Policymaking Graduate

Indiana Autism Coalition Co-Secretary www.inautismcoalition.org

Monica

DisAbility News & Views Radio Show
www.disabilitynewsradio.com

Started an agency called Power Advocates which provides training to parents, and individual consulting to assist with parents of children with disability to receive Free and Appropriate Public Education (FAPE).

Monica says, "While Alexander and I began sharing our story about Asperger's Syndrome and advocacy help with the media in 1999, it was the beginning of being voices for so many others on TV, radio and in newspapers. Because of the lack of the autism awareness and need for autism research, I started the first walk for autism in Buffalo, New York in 2002, called 'Buffalo Walk FAR for NAAR.' Together with seven other committed and caring parents, our first walk had over 3,300 people attend and we raised $100,000 for autism research. It brought a community of people together and autism was officially on the minds of people here. Again in 2003, I co-chaired the walk for autism which was as successful as the year before. As I work full-time at the University at Buffalo, I knew the time I had spent for the past two years as a volunteer for autism had to stop. I had to let go of this and get back to my life with my family and let the torch be carried by others."

"This past year, I wanted to get back to an area I had experienced in – the media, being on the radio. I saw the void there was for people with disabilities and felt a real calling to start my own radio show. It was six months ago that '*DisAbility News & Views Radio Show*' first aired on WXRL Radio 1300 AM, the first live talk hour talk show which focuses on disabilities every Sunday. I have had the opportunity to interview amazing people who continue to inspire me, like my son Alexander. In fact, Alex recently hosted a "Kid's Only" radio show and interviewed Diane Bubel of The Bubel Aiken Foundation. He did a fabulous job! My hope is that the radio show will educate and inspire listeners on the air and on the internet each week, and the radio show will be syndicated so that listeners across the country can call in and share too."

JoAnne

Program Director, Autism & Related Disabilities Gym Program, Inc., Winter Garden, Florida (407) 740-3500 "Enable, Not Disable" — www.autismgym.org

In 2000, JoAnne went to the local rec center and asked to have one hour, one night a week to start a gym program for autistic and related disabilities kids so that they could play and interact with others. They granted her wish along with equipment too! Now they are 180 families strong and a non-profit organization! JoAnne says, "Anyone can start a program like this, all you need to do is ask. There are people willing to help and that care. I urge all parents to start a program like this!"

The Jim Beech Recreational Facility in Ocoee, Florida should be commended for their gracious efforts in accommodating a "Mom with an idea!"

More Heartfelt Thoughts

Autism ~ Heartfelt Thoughts from Fathers is coming soon!
Any Father's who want to contribute, please contact AutismThoughts@yahoo.com

Contributions for ***Autism ~ Heartfelt Thoughts from Family & Friends*** are also being accepted. This includes but is not limited to: Brothers and Sisters, Grandparents, Caregivers, and Teachers. Contact Judy@AutismThoughts.com

or contact:
Autism Enhancement Publishing
PO Box 3141
Olathe, KS 66063

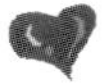

Forgiveness

I struggled with the word Forgiveness for many years. I know that forgiveness is a process in life, something forgiven today may need to be forgiven again tomorrow. I recently was feeling really stuck on this and when I asked my friend Barb about it, she recommended this book called, ***The Little Soul and the Sun*** - A Children's Parable adapted from Conversations with God, by Neale Donald Walsch. I wanted to share this with you because it had a profound affect on me and feel it may touch you also.

~Judy